Nitroglycerin 9

Nitroglycerin 9

Nitrates and Mobility

9th Hamburg Symposium

Editor
T. Meinertz

W DE G

Walter de Gruyter
Berlin · New York 2000

This book contains 30 figures and 13 tables.

The English translation of the articles originally written in German and the German translation of the articles originally written in English was carried out by Dr. Peter Reuter.

Die Deutsche Bibliothek – Cataloging-in-Publication Data

Nitroglycerin 9 : nitrates and mobility / 9th Hamburg Symposium. Ed. T. Meinertz. - Berlin ; New York : de Gruyter, 1999
Dt. Ausgabe. u.d.T.: Nitroglycerin IX
ISBN 3-11-016776-X

Medical science is constantly developing. Research and clinical experience expand our knowledge, especially with regard to treatment and medication. For dosages and applications mentioned in this work, the reader may rely on the authors, editors and publishers having taken great pains to ensure that these indications reflect the standard of knowledge at the time this work was completed.
Nevertheless, all users are requested to check the package leaflet of the medication, in order to determine for themselves whether the recommendations given for the dosages or the likely contraindications differ from those given in this book. This is especially true for medication which is seldom used or has recently been put on the market and for medication whose application has been restricted by the German Ministry of Health.

Copy-editing and typesetting: K. Handwerker, Wissenschafts-Lektorat & DTP Service, Berlin.
Printing: Gerike GmbH, Berlin. – Binding: Lüderitz & Bauer, Berlin.
Printed in Germany

Editor

Prof. Dr. T. Meinertz

Medizinische Klinik
Universitätskrankenhaus Eppendorf
Martinistraße 52
D-20246 Hamburg
Deutschland

List of Contributors

Prof. Dr. S. P. Glasser

School of Public Health
1300 South 2nd Street, Suite 300
Minneapolis, MN 55454
USA

Prof. Dr. E. Jähnchen

Herz-Zentrum Bad Krozingen
Klinische Pharmakologie
Südring 15
D-79189 Bad Krozingen
Deutschland

Dres. I. and G. Kruck

Asperger Straße 48
D-7140 Ludwigsburg
Deutschland

Prof. Dr. W. Langosch

Herz-Zentrum Bad Krozingen
Klinische Pharmakologie
Südring 15
D-79189 Bad Krozingen
Deutschland

Prof. Dr. P. Mathes

Rehabilitationszentrum
München GmbH
Carl-Wery-Straße 26
D-81739 München
Deutschland

Prof. Dr. A. Mülsch

Klinikum der
Johann-Wolfgang-Goethe-Universität
Institut für Kardiovaskuläre
Physiologie
Theodor-Stern-Kai 7
D-60590 Frankfurt/Main
Deutschland

Prof. Dr. J. O. Parker

Department of Cardiovascular
Laboratory
Kingston General Hospital
Kingston, Ontario K7L 2V7
Canada

Prof. Dr. J. Scholze

Charité
Medizinische Poliklinik
Luisenstraße 11-13
D-10098 Berlin
Deutschland

Contents

Introduction

The medical history of nitrates dates back more than 130 years. It all began with the discovery of the antianginal efficacy of nitroglycerin in 1867 (Brunton 1867). Similar observations had been reported by the British physician Alfred Field in 1858. After a series of experiments on himself, he successfully treated a female patient with angina pectoris symptoms and assigned an "antispasmodic" power to the substance. However, the true mechanism of nitrate action remained unclear for the time being.

A monograph published by Sir Thomas Lewis in 1933 mentioned the positive effect of nitroglycerin on dilation of the coronaries as well as the improved myocardial oxygen supply after nitroglycerin application (Lewis 1933). The preload reducing effect of nitrates and the decrease in myocardial oxygen requirement was reported by Gorlin et al. in 1959 (Gorlin et al. 1959).

In 1980 Furchgott and Zawadski (Furchgott et al. 1980) discovered that the vasodilating efficacy of vasodilators depends upon the presence of normal endothelium (endothelial cells). In 1986 Furchgott came to the conclusion that the endothelial factor which produces vasorelaxation, the so-called EDRF, could be nitric oxide (NO) (Furchgott 1988). At around the same time Ignarro et al. (1988) concluded that EDRF was identical with NO or some closely related derivative of it. The pharmacologist Ferid Murad (Houston, Texas) had been working on how nitroglycerin accomplishes vasodilation. In 1977 he found that NO release from nitroglycerin played the most important part. Murad was fascinated by the fact that such a simple gas molecule can regulate cellular functions. After more than one hundred years of therapeutic experience, these results explained the mechanisms of nitrate action.

The importance of the work and discoveries of Furchgott, Ignarro and Murad was emphasized in 1998 when the Nobel prize for medicine was awarded to them. This award clearly demonstrates that even after 130 years nitrates and their effects are still of immediate interest and of outstanding scientific importance. Nitrates have surprised us in the past and they will continue to do so in the future.

However, this book on nitroglycerin is less concerned with basic research than with the clinical use of nitrates. The underlying theme is "Nitrates and Mobility".

What is the importance of exercise therapy for the long term prognosis of patients with coronary heart disease and what role can nitrates play in it?

What is the usefulness of prophylactic application of nitrates?

These are just two topics of this book underscoring the importance of physical activity for patients with angina pectoris. Patients with coronary artery disease quite rightly expect to keep or regain as much quality of life and social integration as possible.

We must not forget to mention the "Nitrolingual Prize" which again was awarded during the 9th Hamburg Nitroglycerin Symposium. Extracts from the prize-winning work of Dr. M. Brückmann can be found in the penultimate chapter of the book. The lectures of the 9th Hamburg Nitroglycerin Symposium 1999 were used as basis for this book.

On behalf of lecturers and organizers of the symposium I would like to invite you to use this book as a source of information, as well as reference book.

T. Meinertz

Endothelial function and nitric oxide (NO): central role in vascular function and protection

A. Mülsch

Introduction

The endothelium, a single-layered, continuous cell sheet lining the luminal vessel wall, separates intravascular (blood) and interstitial compartments. Based on cell count (6 x 10^{13}), mass (1.5 kg), and surface area (1,000 m^2) the endothelium can be looked at as an autonomous organ [24, 16]. For a long time the endothelium was regarded as just being a passive barrier between blood and extravascular space (e.g. for maintenance of the intravascular colloid-osmotic pressure). With the discovery of prostacyclin and other endothelial prostanoids [52] it became apparent for the first time that the endothelium enables communication between intravascular space, vessel wall and tissues via autocrine (intracellular), epicrine (mediated by the endothelial surface), and paracrine (through release of mediators) signals, and thereby exerts an essential homeostatic function. Thus, by release or presentation of signal molecules the endothelium regulates blood coagulation, vessel tone, adhesion and transendothelial migration of monocytes, neovascularization and proliferation of vascular wall cells (Fig. 1). Vasodilating, vasoconstricting, chemotactic, mitogenic, hemostatic, and inflammatory factors as well as factors mediating cell contact are involved (Tab. 1). Due to its pleiotropic actions (see below) NO plays a prominent role in endothelial function compared with other endothelial autocoids. However, endothelial function is also influenced by external factors. For instance, nitric oxide formation is modulated not only by circulating hormones (estrogen), cytokines and released cell products (nucleotides, growth factors), but also by mechanical factors such as endothelial shearing forces generated by the blood flow, pulsatile stretch of the vessel wall, and vascular wall tension. Failure or deficient regulation of these complex endothelial functions can be found in a number of acute and chronic cardiovascular disorders such as atherosclerosis, thromboses, diabetes, and hypertension.

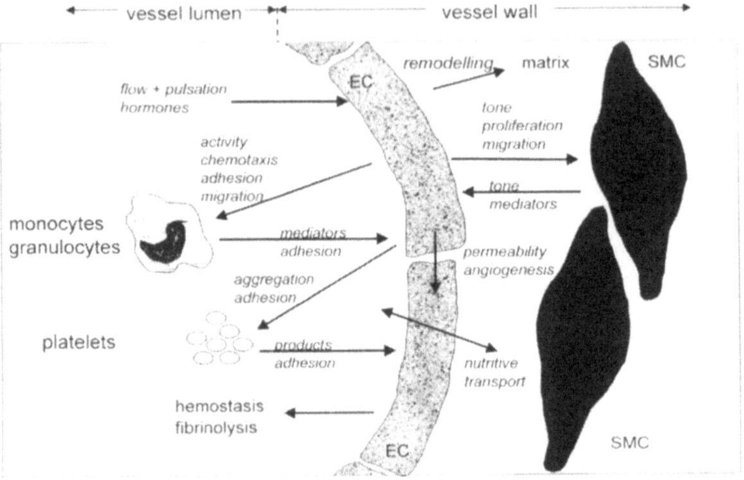

Fig. 1 The endothelium as a regulator of vascular homeostasis.
EC = endothelial cell. SMC = smooth muscle cell. The diagram depicts the interactions between endothelial cells and their environment. For details see text.

Endothelial nitric oxide (NO)

Discovery of endothelium-derived relaxing factor (EDRF) by Furchgott [30] and its subsequent identification as nitric oxide (NO) by Ignarro, Furchgott and Moncada [29, 38] created a new molecular approach towards an understanding of the role of the endothelium in vascular homeostasis. Although the vasodilating properties of NO had been known since 1977 [3, 15, 83, reviewed in 63] the discovery that the volatile gas NO is being produced in the mammalian organism by enzymatic cleavage of L-arginine and is acting as pleiotropic signal molecule came as a surprise. Three isoforms of NO-forming

Table 1 Endothelial signal molecules

signal molecule	acronym/ formula	signal pathway
vasodilators:		
endothelium-derived relaxing factor/ nitric oxide	EDRF/NO	paracrine and autocrine
prostacyclin	PGI_2	paracrine and autocrine
endothelium-derived hyperpolarizing factor	EDHF	paracrine and autocrine
C-type natriuretic peptide	CNP	paracrine and autocrine
bradykinin	Bk	autocrine
vasoconstrictors:		
superoxide anion radical	O_2^-	autocrine and epicrine
endothelin-1	ET-1	paracrine and autocrine
angiotensin II	AT-II	paracrine and autocrine
bradykinin	Bk	paracrine
thromboxane A_2	TxA_2	paracrine
hydroperoxyeicosatetraenoic acids	HPETE	paracrine and autocrine
integrins:		
intercellular adhesion molecule-1	ICAM-1	epicrine
vascular adhesion molecule-1	VCAM-1	epicrine
endothelial-leukocyte adhesion molecule-1	E-selectin/ ELAM-1	epicrine
chemokines:		
monocyte chemoattractant protein-1	MCP-1	paracrine
cytokines:		
interleukins	IL-1	paracrine and autocrine
tumor necrosis factor	TNF-α	paracrine and autocrine
growth factors:		
vascular permeability factor/ endothelial growth factor	VPF/VEGF	paracrine and autocrine
transforming growth factor β	TGFβ	paracrine and autocrine
coagulation factors:		
von-Willebrand-factor	vWF/factor VIII	epicrine/paracrine
tissue plasminogen activator	PA	paracrine
plasminogen activator inhibitor	PAI	paracrine

enzymes have been found so far, neuronal (I), macrophagocytic or inducible (II), and endothelial (III) nitric oxide synthase (NOS) [65]. These isoenzymes resemble the cytochrome P450 system, however, the heme-containing oxidase domain and the flavin-containing reductase domain form one peptide strand [9]. In addition they require tetrahydrobiopterin as cofactor. NO is formed in a NADPH dependent reaction involving the guanidino-N atom of arginine and an activated O_2 molecule.

The endothelial isoform (NOS III; EC 1.14.13.39) can be activated by receptor-dependent agonists such as bradykinin and acetylcholine, and, more importantly, by physical stimulation (fluid shear stress, pulsatile stretch) (Fig. 2). Receptor stimulation leads to transient enzyme activation via increased intracellular Ca^{2+} and binding of calmodulin [10]; shear stress induces NO formation by activation of protein kinase B and phosphorylation of a serine moiety of nitric oxide synthase [18] (Fig. 2). The latter mechanism is physiologically dominant in conductance and resistance vessels. Independent of acute modulation NO formation can be influenced in the long term by changes in the expression of NOS III. Results from cell and animal studies indicate that the vasoprotective effects of estrogens [13] and of physical exercise [84] are due to a transcriptional upregulation of NOS III [26, 94, 100].

Molecular mechanism of NO action

The diversity of the biological actions of nitric oxide is a result of its high membrane permeability, which enables a rapid diffusion across several cell layers [41], and of the high number of NO acceptors (a NO-receptor in a classical sense has not been found so far). Table 2 gives a short but incomplete overview. Important ubiquitous acceptors are NO-binding proteins containing ferro-heme (soluble guanylyl cyclase – sGC; cytochrome c oxidase; hemoglobin; myoglobin), and iron-sulfur centres (aconitase, complex I-III of the mitochondrial respiratory chain) which lose their iron component when reacting with NO [34].

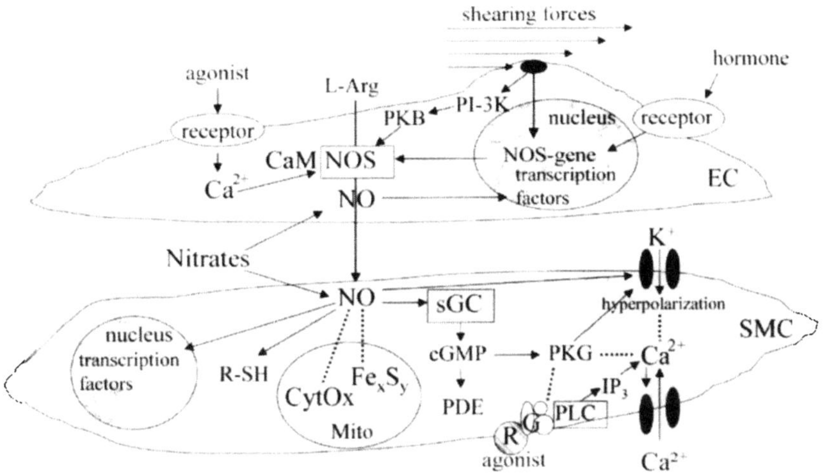

Fig. 2 Activation of endothelial NO synthase and effects of NO.
Upper part: molecular mechanisms of NO synthase (NOS) activation in endothelial cells (EC). For details see text. L-Arg = L-arginine, CaM = calmodulin, PI-3K = phosphatidylinositol 3-kinase, PKB = protein kinase B/akt. Lower part: mechanisms of NO actions on smooth muscle cells (SMC). sGC = soluble guanylyl cyclase, cGMP = cyclic guanosine monophosphate, PKG = protein kinase G, PDE = cGMP-binding phosphodiesterases, R-SH = thiols, CytOx = cytochrome oxidase, Fe_xS_y = iron-sulfur centres in complex I–III of respiratory chain, R = receptor with heterotrimeric G protein, PLC = phospholipase C, IP3 = inositol triphosphate. Arrows indicate the direction of the signal flow, dotted lines symbolize inhibitory signals.

In the cardiovascular system the NO-cGMP signal transduction cascade plays a prominent role (Fig. 2). The binding of NO to the heme-iron of sGC increases the enzyme activity to a level more than a hundred times above the basal activity, and, within a few seconds, leads to a marked increase in the intracellular cGMP concentration [54, 63]. Depending on the cell type further signal transduction is mediated by various effector proteins, among them protein kinases, cyclic nucleotide phosphodiesterases, and cation channels [46].

Table 2 Biologic NO acceptors

acceptor	example	effect
heme	soluble guanylyl cyclase	inhibits vasoconstriction, aggregation, proliferation
	cytochrome oxidase	inhibits mitochondrial oxygen utilization
	cytochrome P450 oxidase	inhibits EDHF-synthesis
	hemoglobin	inactivates NO
	myoglobin	inactivates NO
Fe_xS_y	aconitase	increases cellular iron uptake and mobilization
	mitochondrial complex I–III	inhibits oxidative phosphorylation
Fe-tyrosyl	ribonucleotide reductase	inhibits DNA synthesis
thiol (RSH)	glutathione, cysteine	NO stabilization
	serum albumin	NO stabilization
	caspase	inhibits apoptosis
	glutathione reductase	inhibits glutathione recycling
	glutathione peroxidase	inhibits peroxide detoxification
	G proteins	modulates intracellular signal transduction
	cation channels	modulates membrane potential
ZnS	zinc-finger transcription factors	modulates gene expression

In vascular smooth muscle cells and thrombocytes cGMP activates cGMP-dependent protein kinase Iα which in turn phosphorylates various proteins thus inhibiting vasoconstrictive and pro-aggregatory signal transduction pathways [74]. One target are G-protein-bound receptors [73]. In platelets phosphorylation of the thromboxane A_2-receptor blocks the GTPase activity of the receptor-associated G protein as well as the platelet-activating Ca^{2+} influx [97]. In cultured aortic smooth muscle cells from rats cGMP-dependent protein kinase I phosphorylates and activates a Ca^{2+}-dependent K^+-channel

(B_K-channel) [110]. The induced hyperpolarization of muscle cells diminishes the Ca^{2+} influx induced by contractile agonists thereby inhibiting contraction. Other important NO effects that are mediated by heme-containing and/or iron-sulfur-containing proteins are the inhibition of mitochondrial respiration [47], which regulates the oxygen utilization of tissues, and the regulation of intracellular iron metabolism [101].

Independent of heme and iron-sulfur centers the biological effects of NO are also mediated by thiol compounds. NO and oxidized NO-derivatives (NO^+, HNO_2, NO_2^+, $ONOO^-$) react with low-molecular thiols (cysteine, glutathione) and protein-bound thiol residues (cysteine residues) forming S-nitrosothiols and highly oxidized sulfur oxides [88]. These reactions influence, among other things, the oxygen binding capacity of hemoglobin, the activity of ion channels, G proteins, GSH-dependent enzymes [8] and the so-called zinc-finger transcription factors. S-nitrosation of caspase, a thiol protease, inhibits programmed cell death (apoptosis) of endothelial cells [80]. This mechanism could be of importance for the anti-atherosclerotic effect of NO as increased endothelial apoptosis has been linked to initiation of atherosclerosis [31].

Function of endothelial NO in the cardiovascular system

The most important acute functions of endothelial NO are local regulation of vascular tone, organ perfusion (e.g. heart), oxygen transport and utilization, endothelial permeability and growth, and hemostasis [54]. In the long run endothelial NO protects the vessel wall from atherosclerotic changes by virtue of its anti-apoptotic effect on endothelial cells [31], its growth-inhibiting effect on vascular smooth muscle cells, and its adhesion-inhibiting and anti-inflammatory action on monocytes and granulocytes [108].

Continuous NO release counteracts the basal vessel tone maintained by humoral and neural signals. The importance of this decrease in vessel tone for the regulation of blood pressure becomes apparent when animals are given NOS inhibitors [54] or NOS III is blocked genetically (gene knock-out) [35]. In both cases the mean arterial blood pressure increases significantly. The increased blood pressure in mice with NOS III gene knock-out also shows that neuronal NOS, which is found in the cardiovascular center of the CNS [92] and in non-adrenergic, non-cholinergic (NANC) nerves [91], has only a moderate effect on regulation of vascular tension. Mice lacking the gene for NOS have thickened vessel walls and show paradoxical wall thickening instead of physiologic neovascularization after one-sided carotid ligation [81], a phenomenon attributed to an increased proliferation of vascular muscle cells due to NO deficiency. Changes in flow rate and blood viscosity as well as pulsation influence shearing of the endothelial surface and subsequently NO formation (see chapter on endothelial nitric oxide (NO)). This mechanism, whose molecular basis has been explained recently [18], enables the endothelium to regulate vascular tension and diameter depending on the blood flow, thus reducing compliance of conduction vessels and increasing perfusion of resistance vessels, thereby counteracting an increase in diastolic and systolic blood pressure during increased cardiac output. Similarly, perfusion of distal tissue, e.g. coronaries, can be adjusted according to the perfusion requirements by dilation of proximal vessels [76].

Mode of action of organic nitrates

Organic nitrates, such as nitroglycerin, have been used for treatment and prevention of acute angina pectoris attacks for more than 120 years [64]. The active principle of organic nitrates is NO. It is released from the nitrate moiety via an unknown mechanism that probably involves cytochrome P450-type enzymes [56] and induces vasorelaxation by activating soluble guanylyl cyclase (see above, [63]). This metabolic process is found in endothelial cells and smooth muscle cells of many vessel types [23], however, it is yet undetermined in which cell type the metabolism for the relaxation of smooth muscle cells takes place. Although NO permeates cell membranes easily [41] it is possible that NO released from organic nitrates has an autocrine effect, i.e. its action is limited to the cells it is released in. This would mean that NO released within the endothelium primarily effects endothelial functions, e.g. the macromolecule permeability of the endothelial monolayer [20] and the expression of adhesion and chemotactic proteins [108], whereas NO released within smooth muscle cells primarily inhibits contraction and proliferation of these cells. This also leads to the conclusion that

1. pharmacokinetics and bioavailability of NO generated by endothelial nitric oxide synthase differ from those of NO derived from organic nitrates,
2. the effects of NO derived from organic nitrates on smooth muscle are independent of the endothelial metabolism of nitrates.

However, endothelium derived NO could modulate the efficacy of NO acting on vascular smooth muscle. It has been known for some time that the potency of organic nitrates and of exogenous NO is diminished by the endothelium [75]. It has been shown that this desensitization of vascular smooth muscle is due to endothelial NO formation [53] and cannot be observed with other vasodilators (prostacyclin, papaverine), i.e. it is specific for nitrovasodilators. As desensitization of the cGMP-dependent signal transduction system can be ruled out, it is assumed that soluble guanylyl cyclase is desensitized by endothelial NO itself [53]. Indeed, there seems to exist an inverse correlation between the sensitivity of different vessel types to nitrovasodilators and the rate of NO formation in these vessels [48]. As a matter of fact an increased NO sensitivity of sGC can be detected in homogenates of rat aorta if the vessels are de-endothelialized or the NOS is inhibited prior to homogenization (Fig. 3). The molecular mechanism for this acute sensitization is currently unclear. An important therapeutic consequence of this mechanism could be the preferred action of organic nitrates on vessel segments with missing or dysfunctional endothelium (see below), e.g. coronary segments with early-arteriosclerotic lesions [77]. The anti-vasospastic efficacy of nitroglycerin after PTCA could also be due to an increased NO sensitivity of the vascular muscle [50].

Endothelial dysfunction

The term endothelial dysfunction (ED) cannot be defined exactly as it describes different dysfunctional states depending on the endothelial function it relates to and the underlying disorder. Patients with coronary endothelial dys-

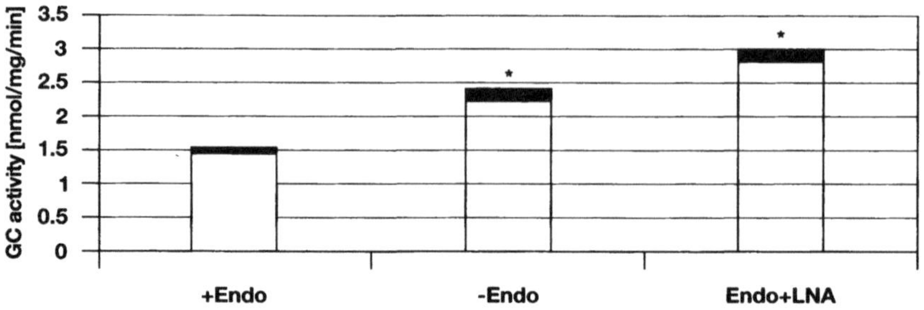

Fig. 3 NO sensitization of soluble guanylyl cyclase through de-endothelialization or inhibition of endothelial NO synthase. Isolated rat aortas, with either intact endothelium (+Endo), or mechanically removed endothelium (-Endo), or after 90 minutes incubation with endothelial NOS inhibitor (N^G-nitro-L-arginine-, LNA, 300 μM), were homogenized and the sodium nitroprusside-stimulated (SNP, 100 μM) activity of sGC in protein extract (10 μg) was determined during 10 minutes (nmol cGMP/min/mg protein). The columns represent median values + SD (n=3) from one representative experiment. Similar results were obtained in two other experiments. Endothelium removal and inhibition of NOS increase significantly (*, $p < =.05$; ANOVA) the SNP-stimulated GC activity.

function and early or advanced atherosclerosis show an increased formation of endothelial vasoconstrictors (angiotensin II, endothelin) [44, 45, 109]. In patients with unstable angina pectoris endothelin was detected in the atherosclerotic tissue of the stenosis [109]. Additionally an increased vasoconstrictor sensitivity of the vascular smooth muscle was reported for ED induced by nitrate tolerance [33]. Furthermore ED is associated with a loss of relaxation after stimulation with endothelium-dependent vasodilators [12]. As a matter of fact these deficiencies can be proven by provocative tests in the early stages of atherosclerosis in patients with the classical risk factors smoking, adiposity, arterial hypertension, diabetes, and hypercholesterolemia (Fig. 4), even before morphologic changes of the vascular wall become apparent. [11, 102]. For example, in coronaries and forearm arteries with dysfunctional endothelium acetylcholine elicits a vasoconstriction (via direct stimulation of muscarinergic acetylcholine receptor of smooth muscle cells) instead of vasodilation [106]. Paradoxical coronary vasoconstriction could also be shown for other more physiologic stimulants of endothelium-dependent relaxation, such as mental stress, cold pressor test, catecholamine infusion, and increased flow [reviewed in 86]. However, there are differences in the degree of the paradoxical vessel response depending on the severity of the dysfunction [107].

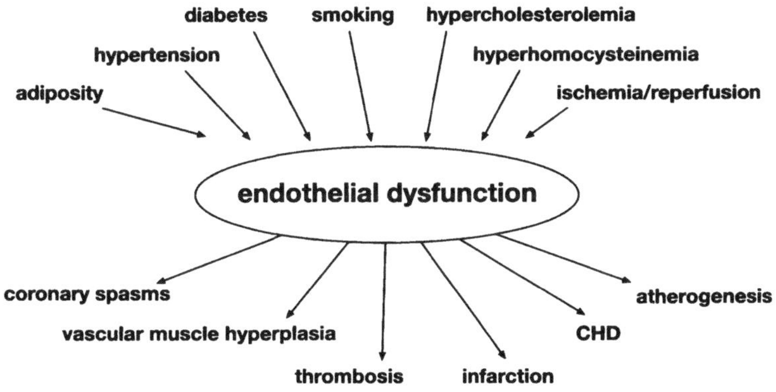

Fig. 4 Causes and consequences of endothelial dysfunction.
The upper part of the diagram lists conditions that potentially promote or cause endothelial dysfunction. The lower part lists potential pathologic consequences.

Reduced NO bioavailability in ED

Originally it was assumed EDRF/NO formation would be reduced in ED [25]. However, it could be shown that NO formation in the vascular wall, determined by the stable NO metabolites NO_2^-/NO_3^-, is normal or even increased [51, 66]. This apparent contradiction was solved when studies by Harrison on rabbits with hypercholesterolemia [68] and Münzel on rabbits with nitrate tolerance [60, 62] showed that in these cases of ED the bioavailability of NO is restricted by increased formation of superoxide radicals (O_2^-) in endothelial and/or smooth muscle cells. The in vivo concentration of O_2^--radicals in human vessels cannot be determined directly, but there is reliable indirect evidence that in patients with ED of different pathogenesis (hypertension, hypercholesterolemia, diabetes, hyperhomocysteinemia, nitrate tolerance) there is an increased inactivation of endothelial NO by O_2^-. This hypothesis is supported by the improvement of ED or the morphologic changes accompanying ED (e.g. vascular wall thickening) with antioxidant therapy [32, 40, 67, 90], as well as the increase in O_2^--metabolites (nitrotyrosine, see below) in ED [5, 87].

Superoxide anion radical

O_2^- is a reactive and toxic oxygen radical that is physiologically formed in low concentrations by one-electron transfer onto oxygen molecules (chemical reduction). The electrons can come from a number of donors (NAD(P)H, xanthine, hypoxanthine) and can be generated by different intracellular reactions [28]. O_2^- dismutates spontaneously generating hydrogen peroxide and molecular oxygen. As this reaction is too slow to allow for a normal cell function it is accelerated by specific enzymes (superoxide dismutases, SOD) [28]. However, the reaction with NO is still three times faster than dismutation with SOD [37], i.e. if O_2^--formation is pathologically elevated, endothelial NO can compete with SOD efficiently.

Depending on the type of endothelial dysfunction different cellular O_2^--sources have been identified: in nitrate-tolerant and hypercholesterolemic rabbits O_2^- is generated by endothelial NADH oxidase, an enzyme similar to the NADPH-oxidase in neutrophilic granulocytes [78]. In this animal model there is also a plasma xanthine oxidase contributing to the endothelial dysfunction [103]. Studies on hypertension and post-infarction models indicate that a NADH oxidase in the vascular smooth muscle is responsible for the ED [4]. Recent studies show that endothelial NO itself is generating O_2^- if the cofactor tetrahydrobiopterin or the substrate L-arginine is missing [14].

Peroxynitrite

The extremely fast reaction with superoxide anion radicals (O_2^-) creating equally short-lived peroxynitrite ($ONOO^-$), appears to be a fundamental mechanism for the limitation of the bioavailability of NO [17, 27]. Peroxynitrite rearranges spontaneously into biologically inactive nitrate (NO_3^-) which is then excreted. Yet, peroxynitrite has its own biologic action spectrum: it can nitrate tyrosine groups of proteins leading to interference with tyrosine kinase-dependent and G-protein-dependent signal transduction pathways [42], inhibit prostacyclin synthesis [111], and block activity of manganese-containing mitochondrial superoxide dismutase (Mn-SOD) [49] leading to an increase in the mitochondrial O_2^--concentration and subsequent damage to the mitochondria [105]. Peroxynitrite also induces in vitro inhibition of sGC, yet, the biologic significance of this phenomenon is unclear [95]. Increased nitrotyrosine formation can be found in arteriosclerosis [5] and nitrate tolerance [87].

To sum it up it can be said that increased inactivation of endothelial NO by O_2^- is a major factor in development of endothelial dysfunction for a variety of underlying disorders. However, this mechanism does not only interfere with the regulation of the vascular tone (hypertension), but also with all other homeostatic and protective functions of the endothelium (antithrombotic effect, anti-atherosclerotic potential, and so forth).

Therapy of endothelial dysfunction

NO substitution and endothelium protection with organic nitrates

The pharmacological profile of organic nitrates is primarily based on a preload reduction through venous pooling and a dilation of the large coronaries. These mechanisms reduce myocardial workload, reduce the oxygen requirement, and economize cardiac work [1]. Myocardial resistance vessels are not affected, thus there is no steal phenomenon. Reduction of the afterload (diastolic arterial pressure) requires high doses, whereas the compliance of arterial conductance vessels is already improved at low doses [1]. Based on this pharmacodynamic profile nitrates are indicated in acute myocardial infarction, acute left heart failure, hypertensive crisis, as well as in the prophylaxis of angina pectoris, during coronary angiography, and for blood pressure reduction prior to cardiovascular surgery (see following chapters).

Organic nitrates can compensate for the acute lack of NO in coronary endothelial dysfunction, thus offering effective treatment for exercise-induced angina pectoris or angina due to vasospasm [36].

Yet, it is still unclear whether organic nitrates can substitute for all functions of endothelial NO. So far there are no controlled studies proving an anti-atherosclerotic, anti-apoptotic, anti-adhesive, or antiproliferative efficacy of organic nitrates in normal therapeutic doses. Anti-aggregatory effects can be shown in animal studies [19], however, it is not clear whether nitrates used in hemodynamically effective doses inhibit platelets directly, or whether endothelial prostacyclin mediates the effect [82].

Recently a study on hypercholesterolemic rabbits pointed at a possible endothelium-protective effect of long-term application of low-dose (hemodynamically ineffective) nitrates. In this study the decrease in endothelium-dependent relaxation induced by high-cholesterol diet was offset by concomitant administration of organic nitrates [39]. Clinical studies will have to show if this beneficial effect can also be achieved in hypercholesterolemic and atherosclerotic patients.

Increase in the bioavailability of endothelial NO

New therapeutic strategies for ED should, among other things, try to improve the bioavailability of endothelial NO, i.e., reduce O_2^--formation. Animal as well as clinical studies show that this goal can be achieved by low-cholesterol diet [69], antilipidemics [22, 93], antioxidants such as vitamin C [32, 90], vitamin E [67, 98] (HOPE study with vitamin E was negative!), and probucol [85], administration of cell membrane-permeable SOD [55], L-arginine infusion to increase the substrate level for NO synthesis [21], and, probably, tetrahydrobiopterin (NOS cofactor) infusion [14]. Some types of ED are marked by an increased ACE activity in the vessel wall and an elevated plasma AT II level leading to an increased O_2^--formation. In these cases a reduction in vascular O_2^--formation and restitution of the normal endothelial function can be achieved with ACE inhibitors [33, 71] (clinically proven in the TREND, BANFF, and HOPE studies) and angiotensin-receptor antagonists

[62]. Hydralazine, a long used antihypertensive agent, inhibits endothelial NADH-oxidase thus increasing the bioavailability of endothelial NO [61]. The above-mentioned studies prove that ED can potentially be reversed.

Exploitation of the NO mechanism with other cardiovascular agents

There are indications from animal and cell studies that NO is directly or indirectly linked to the efficacy of a number of drugs that are not nitrovasodilators (nitrates, sodium nitroprusside, molsidomine). ACE inhibitors not only block the formation of the vasoconstrictor angiotensin II, but also the breakdown of bradykinin thus increasing formation of endothelial NO [104]. ACE inhibitors also increase NO formation by blocking internalization of bradykinin receptors after stimulation by bradykinin [6]. Nifedipine and other dihydropyridine type calcium antagonists stimulate endothelial NO formation via a yet unknown mechanism [7]. HMG-CoA-reductase inhibitors (statins), used to lower lipid levels, increase expression of the endothelial NO synthase [43]. Currently there are first models for gene therapy to increase local expression of NO synthase. One approach is to use a vector to implant a NO synthase gene (endothelial or inducible NOS) into the vessel wall and to induce transient expression of the gene, hoping that this will help to bridge the critical period between endothelial damage by catheter ablation and formation of a functional neo-endothelium [96]. An overview on the various therapeutic possibilities is given in Fig. 5.

Improve NO sensitivity of vascular smooth muscle and platelets

Independent from endothelial dysfunction vascular dysfunction can be caused by smooth muscle dysfunction [2]. Apart from the increased vasoconstrictor sensitivity already mentioned above, smooth muscle dysfunction can be due to a reduced expression or diminished NO sensitivity of soluble guanylyl cyclase [4, 72, 79]. Drugs acting via an increased bioavailability of endothelial NO or exogenous application of NO (nitrovasodilators) will be of no use in these cases, as NO cannot achieve vasodilation. A better therapeutic approach is to increase NO efficacy in smooth muscle cells by use of NO sensitizers. NO sensitizers are a new group of sGC activators which do not produce NO but lead to a selective increase in the NO-sensitivity of this key enzyme of NO-dependent signal transduction. One cardinal substance is YC-1 which potentiates the vasodilatory, antihypertensive and anti-aggregatory effects of nitrovasodilators at low concentration exerting no effect on its own [57, 89].

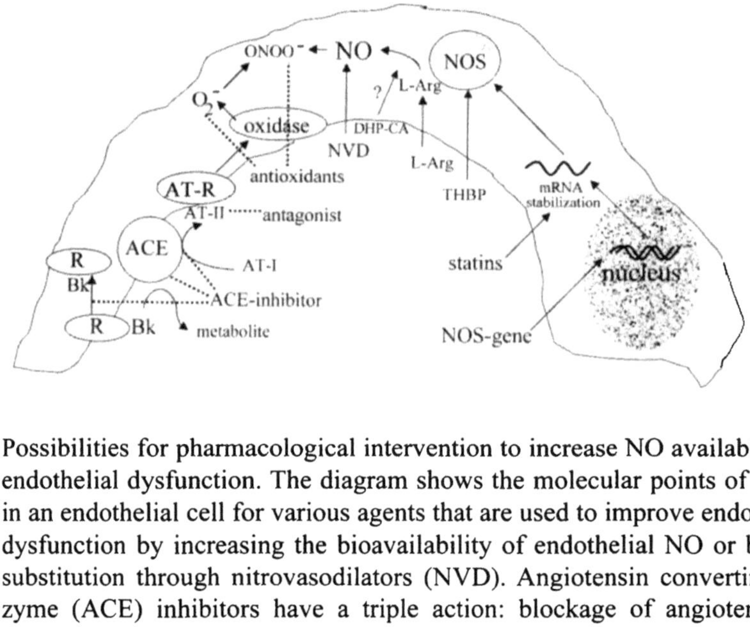

Fig. 5 Possibilities for pharmacological intervention to increase NO availability in endothelial dysfunction. The diagram shows the molecular points of action in an endothelial cell for various agents that are used to improve endothelial dysfunction by increasing the bioavailability of endothelial NO or by NO substitution through nitrovasodilators (NVD). Angiotensin converting enzyme (ACE) inhibitors have a triple action: blockage of angiotensin II (AT II) formation, of bradykinin (Bk) breakdown, and of internalization of bradykinin receptor (R). Angiotensin-receptor (AT-R) antagonists block AT binding. Antioxidants reduce superoxide (O_2^-) and peroxynitrite ($ONOO^-$) load by cellular oxidases. Dihydropyridine type calcium antagonists (DHP-CA), L-arginine (L-Arg), and tetrahydrobiopterin (THBP) increase NOS activity. HMG-CoA-reductase inhibitors (statins) stabilize NOS-mRNA thus increasing NOS expression. This can also be achieved by transfection of the NOS gene.

Summary and outlook

Nitric oxide contributes considerably to the vasorelaxing, anti-aggregatory, anti-proliferative, and anti-atherosclerotic action of endothelial cells. In endothelial dysfunction bioavailability of NO is diminished by vascular O_2^- formation. Therapy of ED aims at increasing the NO availability with the help of exogenous NO donors (nitrates), reducing O_2^--formation with antioxidants, blocking the O_2^--generating signal transduction cascade, and increasing the NO sensitivity of target cells at the same time. Therefore, it can be assumed that bioavailability and biologic action of endothelial NO will remain therapeutic targets for the future.

References

[1] Abrams, J.: Use of nitrates in ischemic heart disease. Curr. Probl. Cardiol. 17 (1992) 481–542.

[2] Adams, M.R., J. Robinson, R. McCredie et al.: Smooth muscle dysfunction occurs independently of impaired endothelium-dependent dilation in adults at risk of atherosclerosis. J. Am. Coll. Cardiol. 32 (1998) 123–127.

[3] Arnold, W.P., C.K. Mittal, S. Katsuki, F. Murad: Nitric oxide activates guanylate cyclase and increases guanosine 3',5'-cyclic monophosphate levels in various tissue preparations. Proc. Natl. Acad. Sci. U.S.A. 74 (1977) 3203–3207.

[4] Bauersachs, J., A. Bouloumie, A. Mülsch et al.: Vasodilator dysfunction in aged spontaneously hypertensive rats: changes in NO synthase III and soluble guanylyl cyclase expression, and in superoxide anion production. J. Cardiovasc. Res. 37 (1998) 772–779.

[5] Beckman, J.S., Z.Y. Ye, P.G. Anderson et al.: Extensive nitration of protein tyrosines in human atherosclerosis detected by immunohistochemistry. Hoppe-Seylers Z. Physiol. Chem. 375 (1994) 81–88.

[6] Benzing, T., I. Fleming, A. Blaukat et al.: Angiotensin-converting enzyme inhibitor ramiprilat interferes with the sequestration of the B2 kinin receptor within the plasma membrane of native endothelial cells. Circulation 99 (1999) 2034–2040.

[7] Berkels, R., W. Klaus, M. Boller et al.: The calcium modulator nifedipine exerts its antiaggregatory property via a nitric oxide mediated process.Thrombos. Haemostas. 72 (1994) 309–312.

[8] Boese, M., M.A. Keese, K. Becker et al.: Inhibition of glutathione reductase by dinitrosyl-iron complex. J. Biol. Chem. 272 (1997) 21767–21773.

[9] Bredt, D.S., P.H. Hwang, C. Glatt et al.: Cloned and expressed nitric oxide synthase structurally resembles cytochrome P450 reductase. Nature 351 (1991) 714–718.

[10] Busse, R., A. Mülsch: Calcium-dependent nitric oxide synthesis in endothelial cytosol is mediated by calmodulin. FEBS Lett. 265 (1990) 133–136.

[11] Celermayer, D.S., K.E. Sorensen, V.M. Gooch et al.: Noninvasive detection of endothelial dysfunction in children and adults at risk of atherosclerosis. Lancet 340 (1992) 1111–1115.

[12] Cohen, R.A., K.M. Zitnay, C.C. Haudenschild et al.: Loss of selective endothelial cell vasoactive functions caused by hypercholesterolemia in pig coronary arteries. Circ. Res. 63 (1988) 903–910.

[13] Collins, P., G.M.C. Rosano, P.M. Sarrel et al.: 17β-estradiol attenuates acetylcholine-induced coronary artery constriction in women but not in men with coronary artery disease. Circulation 92 (1995) 24–30.

[14] Cosentino, F., S. Patton, L.V. d'Uscio et al.: Tetrahydrobiopterin alters superoxide and nitric oxide release in prehypertensive rats. J. Clin. Invest. 101 (1998) 1530–1537.

[15] Craven, P.A., F.R. DeRubertis: Restoration of the responsiveness of purified guanylate cyclase to nitrosoguanidine, nitric oxide, and related activators by heme and hemeproteins. Evidence for the involvement of paramagnetic nitrosyl-heme complex in enzyme activation. J. Biol. Chem. 253 (1978) 8433–8443.

[16] Cryer, A.: Scale and diversity of interactions at the vascular endothelium. In: Cryer, A. (Hrsg.): Biochemical interactions at the endothelium, S. 1–3. Elsevier, Amsterdam/New York/Oxford 1983.

[17] Darley-Usmar, V.M., H. Wiseman, B. Halliwell: Nitric oxide and oxygen radicals: a question of balance. FEBS Lett. 369 (1995) 131–135.

[18] Dimmeler, S., I. Fleming, B. Fissithaler et al.: Activation of nitric oxide synthase in endothelial cells by Akt-dependent phosphorylation. Nature 399 (1999) 601–605.

[19] Diodati, J., P. Theroux, J.G. Latour: Effects of nitroglycerin at therapeutic doses on platelet aggregation in unstable angina pectoris and myocardial infarction platelets, vasoconstriction, and nitroglycerin during arterial wall injury: a new antithrombotic role for an old drug: importance of adequate heparin dosage in arterial angioplasty in a porcine model. Am. J. Cardiol. 78 (1988) 654–660.

[20] Draijer, R., D.E. Atsma, A. van der Laarse et al.: cGMP and nitric oxide modulate thrombin-induced endothelial permeability. Regulation via different pathways in human umbilical vein endothelial cells. Circ. Res. 76 (1995) 199–208.

[21] Drexler, H., A.M. Zeiher, K. Meinzer et al.: Correction of endothelial dysfunction in coronary microcirculation of hypercholesterolemic patients by L-arginine. Lancet 338 (1991) 1546–1550.
[22] Egashira, K., H.Y. Kai et al.: Reduction of serum cholesterol with pravastatin improves endothelium-dependent coronary vasomotion in patients with hypercholesterolemia. J. Infect. Dis. 172 (1995) 585–588.
[23] Feelisch, M., M. Kelm: Biotransformation of organic nitrates to nitric oxide by vascular smooth muscle and endothelial cells. Biochem. Biophys. Res. Commun. 180 (1991) 286–293.
[24] Fishman, A.P.: Endothelium: a distributed organ with diverse capabilities. Ann. N.Y. Acad. Sci. 401 (1982) 1–8.
[25] Förstermann, U., A. Mügge, U. Alheid et al.: Selective attenuation of endothelium-mediated vasodilation in atherosclerotic human coronary arteries. Circ. Res. 62 (1988) 185–190.
[26] Förstermann, U., H. Kleinert: Nitric oxide synthase: expression and expressional control of the three isoforms. Naunyn-Schmiedebergs Arch. Pharmacol. 352 (1995) 351–364.
[27] Freeman, B.A., C.R. White, H. Gutierrez et al.: Oxygen radical-nitric oxide reactions in vascular diseases. Adv. Pharmacol. 34 (1995) 45–58.
[28] Fridovich, I.: The biology of oxygen radicals. Science 201 (1979) 879–880.
[29] Furchgott, R.F., M.T. Khan, D. Jothianandan: Evidence supporting the proposal that endothelium-derived relaxing factor is nitric oxide. Thromb. Res. 7 (Suppl. 7) (1987) 3 (Abstract).
[30] Furchgott, R.F., J.V. Zawadzki: The obligatory role of endothelial cells in the relaxation of arterial smooth muscle by acetylcholine. Nature 228 (1980) 373–376.
[31] Haendeler, J., A.M. Zeiher, S. Dimmeler: Nitric oxide and apoptosis. Vitam. Horm. 57 (1999) 49–77.
[32] Heitzer, T. J.H. Just, T. Münzel: Antioxidant vitamin C improves endothelial dysfunction in chronic smokers. Circulation 94 (1996) 6–9.
[33] Heitzer, T., H. Just, C. Brockhoff et al.: Long-term nitroglycerin treatment is associated with supersensitivity to vasoconstrictors in men with stable coronary artery disease: prevention by concomitant treatment with captopril. J. Am. Coll. Cardiol. 31 (1998) 83–88.
[34] Henry, Y., M. Lepoivre, J.C. Drapier et al.: EPR characterization of molecular targets for NO in mammalian cells and organelles. FASEB J. 7 (1993) 1124–1134.
[35] Huang, P.L., Z.H. Huang, H. Mashimo et al.: Hypertension in mice lacking the gene for endothelial nitric oxide synthase. Nature 377 (1995) 239–242.
[36] Hütter, P., K. Strein: Nitrattherapie – eine kausale Therapie des Angina pectoris-Syndroms? Fortschr. Med. 106 (1988) 413–416.

[37] Huie, R.E., S. Padjama: The reaction rate of nitric oxide with superoxide. Free Rad. Res. Commun. 18 (1993) 195–199.

[38] Ignarro, L.J., G.M. Buga, K.S. Wood et al.: Endothelium-derived relaxing factor produced and released from artery and vein is nitric oxide. Proc. Natl. Acad. Sci. U.S.A. 84 (1987) 9265–9269.

[39] Kojda, G., D. Stein, E. Kottenberg et al.: In vivo effects of pentaerithrityl-tetranitrate and isosorbide-5-mononitrate on the development of atherosclerosis and endothelial dysfunction in cholesterol-fed rabbits. J. Cardiovasc. Pharmacol. 25 (1995) 763–773.

[40] Kritchevsky, S.B., T. Shimakawa, G.S. Tell et al.: Dietary antioxidants and carotid artery wall thickness. Circulation 92 (1995) 2142–2150.

[41] Lancaster, J.R.: Simulation of the diffusion and reaction of endogenously produced nitric oxide. Proc. Natl. Acad. Sci. U.S.A. 91 (1994) 8137–8141.

[42] Lander, H.M., P.K. Sehajpal, A. Novogrodsky: Nitric oxide signaling: a possible role for G proteins. J. Immunol. 151 (1993) 7182–7187.

[43] Laufs, U., V. La Fata, J. Plutzky et al.: Upregulation of endothelial nitric oxide synthase by HMG CoA reductase inhibitors. Circulation 97 (1998) 1129–1135.

[44] Lerman, A., B.S. Edwards, J.W. Hallett et al.: Circulating and tissue endothelin immunoreactivity in advanced atherosclerosis. N. Engl. J. Med. 325 (1991) 997–1001.

[45] Lerman, A., D.R. Holmes, M.R. Bell et al.: Endothelin in coronary endothelial dysfunction and early atherosclerosis in humans. Circulation 92 (1995) 2426–2431.

[46] Lincoln, T.M., T.L. Cornwell: Intracellular cyclic GMP receptor proteins. FASEB J. 7 (1993) 328–338.

[47] Loke, K.E., P.I. McConnel, J.M. Tuzman et al.: Endogenous endothelial nitric oxide synthase-derived nitric oxide is a physiological regulator of myocardial oxygen consumption. Circ. Res. 84 (1999) 840–845.

[48] Lüscher, T.F.: Endothelium-derived nitric oxide: the endogenous nitrovasodilator in the human cardiovascular system. Eur. Heart J. 12 (Suppl. E) (1991) 2–11.

[49] MacMillan-Crow, L.A., J.P. Crow, J.D. Kerby et al.: Nitration and inactivation of manganese superoxide dismutase in chronic rejection of human renal allografts. Proc. Natl. Acad. Sci. U.S.A. 93 (1996) 11853–11858.

[50] Margolis, J.R., C. Chen: Coronary artery spasm complicating PTCA: role of intracoronary nitroglycerin. Z. Kardiol. 78 (Suppl. 2) (1989) 41–44.

[51] Minor, R.L., P.R. Myers, R. Guerra et al.: Diet-induced atherosclerosis increases the release of nitrogen oxides from rabbit aorta. J. Clin. Invest. 86 (1990) 2109–2116.

[52] Moncada, S., J.R. Vane: Pharmacology and endogenous roles of prostaglandin endoperoxides, thromboxane A2, and prostacyclin. Pharmacol. Rev. 30 (1979) 293–331.

[53] Moncada, S., D.D. Rees, R. Schulz et al.: Development and mechanism of a specific supersensitivity to nitrovasodilators after inhibition of vascular nitric oxide synthesis in vivo. Proc. Natl. Acad. Sci. U.S.A. 88 (1991) 2166–2170.

[54] Moncada, S., A. Higgs: Mechanisms of disease: The L-arginine-nitric oxide pathway. N. Engl. J. Med. 329 (1993) 2002–2012.

[55] Mügge, A., J.H. Elwell, T.E. Peterson et al.: Chronic treatment with polyethylene-glycolated superoxide dismutase partially restores endothelium-dependent vascular relaxations in cholesterol-fed rabbits. Circ. Res. 69 (1991) 1293–1300.

[56] Mülsch, A., P.M. Mordvintcev, E. Bassenge et al.: In vivo spin trapping of glycerol trinitrate-derived nitric oxide in rabbit blood vessels and organs. Circulation 92 (1995) 1876–1882.

[57] Mülsch, A., J. Bauersachs, A. Schäfer et al.: Effect of YC-1, an NO-independent, superoxide-sensitive stimulator of soluble guanylyl cyclase, on smooth muscle responsiveness to nitrovasodilators. Br. J. Pharmacol. 120 (1997) 681–689.

[58] Mülsch, A., S. Klöß: Die lösliche Guanylylcyclase ist ein Peroxynitrit-Rezeptor. Z. Kardiol. 88 (Suppl. 1) (1999) 925 (Abstract).

[59] Münzel, T., A. Giaid, S. Kurz et al.: Evidence for a role of endothelin 1 and protein kinase C in nitroglycerin tolerance. Proc. Natl. Acad. Sci. U.S.A. 92 (1995) 5244–5248.

[60] Münzel, T., H. Sayegh, B.A. Freeman et al.: Evidence for enhanced vascular superoxide production in nitrate tolerance. J. Clin. Invest. 95 (1995) 187–194.

[61] Münzel, T., S. Kurz, S. Rajagopalan: Hydralazine prevents nitroglycerin tolerance by inhibiting activation of a membrane-bound NADH oxidase. A new action for an old drug. J. Clin. Invest. 98 (1996) 1465–1470.

[62] Münzel, T., D.G. Harrison: Evidence for a role of oxygen-derived free radicals and protein kinase C in nitrate tolerance. J. Mol. Med. 75 (1997) 891–900.

[63] Murad, F.: Regulation of cytosolic guanylyl cyclase by nitric oxide: the NO-cyclic GMP signal transduction system. Adv. Pharmacol. 26 (1994) 19–33.

[64] Murrell, W.: Nitroglycerin as a remedy for angina pectoris. Lancet 1 (1879) 80–81.

[65] Nathan, C., Q. Xie: Nitric oxide synthases: Roles, tolls, and controls. Cell 78 (1994) 915–918.

[66] Nava, E., G. Noll, T.F. Lüscher: The increased activity of constitutive nitric oxide synthase in cardiac endothelium in spontaneous hypertension. Circulation 91 (1995) 2310–2313.

[67] Nunes, G.L., K. Robinson, A. Kalynych et al.: Vitamins C and E inhibit O_2^- production in the pig coronary artery. Circulation 96 (1997) 3593–3601.
[68] Ohara, Y., T.E. Peterson, D.G. Harrison: Hypercholesterolemia increases endothelial superoxide anion production. J. Clin. Invest. 91 (1993) 2546–2551.
[69] Ohara, Y., T.E. Peterson, H.S. Sayegh et al.: Dietary correction of hypercholesterolemia in the rabbit normalizes endothelial superoxide anion production. Circulation 92 (1995) 898–903.
[70] Palmer, R.M.J., A.G. Ferridge, S. Moncada: Nitric oxide release accounts for the biological activity of endothelium-derived relaxing factor. Nature 327 (1987) 524–526.
[71] Panza, J.A., A.A. Quyyumi, T.S. Callahan et al.: Effect of antihypertensive treatment on endothelium-dependent vascular relaxation in patients with essential hypertension. J. Am. Coll. Cardiol. 21 (1993) 1145–1151.
[72] Papapetropoulos, A., N. Marczin, M.D. Snead et al.: Smooth muscle cell responsiveness to nitrovasodilators in hypertensive and normotensive rats. Hypertension 23 (1994) 476–484.
[73] Pfeifer, A., B. Nürnberg, S. Kamm et al.: Cyclic GMP-dependent protein kinase blocks pertussis toxin-sensitive hormone receptor signaling pathways in chinese hamster ovary cells. J. Biol. Chem. 270 (1995) 9052–9059.
[74] Pfeifer, A., P. Klatt, S. Massberg et al.: Defective smooth muscle regulation in cGMP kinase I-deficient mice. EMBO J. 17 (1998) 3045–3051.
[75] Pohl, U., R. Busse: Endothelium-derived relaxant factor inhibits effects of nitrocompounds in isolated arteries. Am. J. Physiol. 252 (1987) H307–H313.
[76] Pohl, U., D. Lamontagne, E. Bassenge, R. Busse: Attenuation of coronary autoregulation in the isolated rabbit heart by endothelium-derived nitric oxide. Cardiovasc. Res. 28 (1994) 414–419.
[77] Rafflenbeul, W., E. Bassenge, P.R. Lichtlen: Konkurrenz zwischen endothelabhängiger und Nitroglycerin-induzierter koronarer Relaxation. Z. Kardiol. 78 (Suppl. 2) (1989)
[78] Rajagopalan, S., S. Kurz, T. Münzel et al.: Angiotensin II-mediated hypertension in the rat increases vascular superoxide production via membrane NADH/NADPH oxidase activation. Contributions to alterations in vasomotor tone. J. Clin. Invest. 97 (1996) 1916–1923.
[79] Robinson, B.F., R.J. Dobbs, S. Bayley: Response of forearm resistance vessels to verapamil and sodium nitroprusside in normotensive and hypertensive men: evidence for a functional abnormality of vascular smooth muscle in primary hypertension. Clin Sci. 63 (1982) 33–42.
[80] Rossig, L., B. Fichtlscherer, K. Breitschopf et al.: Nitric oxide inhibits caspase-3 by S-nitrosation in vivo. J. Biol. Chem. 274 (1999) 6823–6826.

[81] Rudic, R.D., E.G. Shesely, N. Maeda et al.: Direct evidence for the importance of endothelium-derived nitric oxide in vascular remodeling. J. Clin. Invest. 101 (1998) 731–736.
[82] Schröder, H., K. Schrör: Organische Nitrate und Thrombozytenfunktion. Hamostasiologie 8 (1988) 90–99.
[83] Schultz, K.D., K. Schultz, G. Schultz: Sodium nitroprusside and other smooth muscle relaxants increase cyclic GMP levels in rat ductus deferens. Nature 265 (1977) 750–751.
[84] Sessa, W.C., K. Pritchard, N. Seyedi et al.: Chronic exercise in dogs increases coronary vascular nitric oxide production and endothelial cell nitric oxide synthase gene expression. Circ. Res. 74 (1994) 349–353.
[85] Simon, B.C., C.C. Haudenschild, R.A. Cohen: Preservation of endothelium-dependent relaxation in atherosclerotic rabbit aorta by probucol. J. Cardiovasc. Pharmacol. 21 (1993) 893–901.
[86] Simon, B.C., B. Noll, B. Maisch: Endotheliale Dysfunktion – eine Bestandsaufnahme und Ansätze zur Therapie. Herz 24 (1999) 62–71.
[87] Skatchkov, M., L. Larina, A. Larin et al.: Urinary nitrotyrosine content as a marker of peroxynitrite-induced tolerance to organic nitrates. J. Cardiovasc. Pharmacol. Ther. 2 (1997) 85–96.
[88] Stamler, J.S., E.J. Toone, S.A. Lipton et al.: (S)NO signals: translocation, regulation, and a consensus motif. Neuron 18 (1997) 691–696.
[89] Teng, C.M., C.C. Wu, F.-N. Ko et al.: YC-1, a nitric oxide-independent activator of soluble guanylate cyclase, inhibits platelet-rich thrombosis in mice. Eur. J. Pharmacol. 320 (1997) 161–166.
[90] Ting, H.H., F.K. Timimi, E.A. Haley et al.: Vitamin C improves endothelium-dependent vasodilation in forearm resistance vessels of humans with hypercholesterolemia. Circulation 95 (1997) 2617–2622.
[91] Toda, N., K. Yoshida, T. Okamura: Analysis of the potentiating action of N^G-nitro-L-arginine on the contraction of the dog temporal artery elicited by transmural stimulation of noradrenergic nerves. Naunyn-Schmiedebergs Arch. Pharmacol. 343 (1991) 221–224.
[92] Togashi, H., I. Sakuma, M. Yoshioka et al.: A central nervous system action of nitric oxide in blood pressure regulation. J. Pharmacol. Exper. Ther. 262 (1992) 343–347.
[93] Treasure, C.B., J.L. Klein, W.S. Weintraub: Beneficial effects of cholesterin-lowering therapy on the coronary endothelium in patients with coronary artery disease. N. Engl. J. Med. 332 (1995) 481–487.
[94] Uematsu, M., Y. Ohara, J.P. Navas et al.: Regulation of endothelial cell nitric oxide synthase mRNA by shear stress. Am. J. Physiol. 269 (1995) C1371–C1378.

[95] Villa, L.M., E. Salas, V. Darley-Usmar et al.: Peroxynitrite induces both vasodilation and impaired vasorelaxation in the isolated perfused rat heart. Proc. Natl. Acad. Sci. U.S.A. 91 (1994) 12383–12387.

[96] Von der Leyen, H.E., G.H. Gibbons, R. Morishita et al.: Gene therapy inhibiting neointimal vascular lesions: in vivo transfer of endothelial cell nitric oxide synthase gene. Proc. Natl. Acad. Sci. U.S.A. 92 (1995) 1137–1141.

[97] Wang, G.R., Y. Zhu, P.V. Halushka et al.: Mechanism of platelet inhibition by nitric oxide: in vivo phosphorylation of thromboxane receptor by cyclic GMP-dependent protein kinase. Proc. Natl. Acad. Sci. U.S.A. 95 (1998) 4888–4893.

[98] Watanabe, H., M. Kakihana, S. Ohtsuka et al.: Randomized, double-blind, placebo-controlled study of supplemental vitamin E on attenuation of the development of nitrate tolerance. Circulation 94 (1996) 503–504.

[99] Weber, A.A, H. Strobach, K. Schrör: Direct inhibition of platelet function by organic nitrates via nitric oxide formation. Eur. J. Pharmacol. 247 (1993) 29–37.

[100] Weiner, C.P., I. Lizasoin, S.A. Baylis et al.: Induction of calcium-dependent nitric oxide synthases by sex hormones. Proc. Natl. Acad. Sci. U.S.A. 91 (1994) 5212–5216.

[101] Weiss, G., B. Goosen, W. Doppler et al.: Translational regulation via iron-resposive elements by the nitric oxide/NO-synthase pathway. EMBO J. 12 (1993) 3651–3657.

[102] Werns, S.W., J.A. Walton, H.H. Hsia et al.: Evidence of endothelial dysfunction in angiographically normal coronary arteries of patients with coronary artery disease. Circulation 79 (1989) 287–291.

[103] White, C.R., V. Darley-Usmar, W.R. Berrington et al.: Circulating plasma xanthine oxidase contributes to vascular dysfunction in hypercholesterolemic rabbits. Proc. Natl. Acad. Sci. U.S.A. 93 (1996) 8745–8749.

[104] Wiemer, G., W. Linz, S. Hatrik et al.: Angiotensin-converting enzyme inhibition alters nitric oxide and superoxide release in normotensive and hypertensive rats. Hypertension 30 (1997) 1183–1190.

[105] Xie, Y.W., P.M. Kaminski, M.S. Wolin: Inhibition of rat cardiac muscle contraction and mitochondrial respiration by endogenous peroxynitrite formation during posthypoxic reoxygenation. Circ. Res. 82 (1998) 891–897.

[106] Zeiher, A.M., H. Drexler, H. Wollschläger et al.: Coronary vasomotion in response to sympathetic stimulation in humans: importance of the functional integrity of the endothelium. J. Am. Coll. Cardiol. 14 (1989) 1181–1190.

[107] Zeiher, A.M., H. Drexler, H. Wollschläger et al.: Modulation of coronary vasomotor tone in humans: Progressive endothelial dysfunction with different early stages of coronary atherosclerosis. Circulation 83 (1991) 391–401.

[108] Zeiher, A.M., B. Fisslthaler, B. Schray-Utz et al.: Nitric oxide modulates the expression of monocyte chemoattractant protein 1 in cultured human endothelial cells. Circ. Res. 76 (1995) 980–986.

[109] Zeiher, A.M., H. Goebel, V. Schachinger et al.: Tissue endothelin-1 immunoreactivity in the active coronary atherosclerotic plaque: a clue to the mechanism of increased vasoreactivity of the culprit lesion in unstable angina. Circulation 91 (1995) 941–947.

[110] Zhou, X.-B., P. Ruth, J. Schlossmann et al.: Protein phosphatase 2A is essential for the activation of Ca^{2+}-activated K^{+}-currents by cGMP-dependent protein kinase in tracheal smooth muscle and chinese hamster ovary cells. J. Biol. Chem. 271 (1996) 19760–19767.

[111] Zou, M., M. Jendral, V. Ullrich: Prostaglandin endoperoxide-dependent vasospasm in bovine coronary arteries after nitration of prostacyclin synthase. Br. J. Pharmacol. 126 (1999) 1283–1292.

Organic nitrates: has the therapeutic potential been exhausted?

E. Jähnchen

Organic nitrates are vasodilators. They achieve vasodilation by release of nitric oxide (NO), which stimulates guanylyl cyclase, thereby leading to formation of cyclic guanosine monophosphate (cGMP), which in turn relaxes vascular smooth muscle.

In contrast to other vasodilators (e.g., hydralazine, calcium channel blockers) organic nitrates primarily act on venous capacitance vessels (in particular, pulmonary and splanchnic vessels), thus reducing the preload. Larger subepicardial coronaries are susceptible to organic nitrates, too [3]. However, peripheral resistance vessels need higher concentration of nitrates before dilating. This vascular selectivity is due to different enzyme patterns for different vascular sites. These enzymes are of importance for the release of nitric oxide from the active principle.

Another selectivity mechanism of organic nitrates is the their preferred action on dysfunctional vascular segments compared to normal vessel segments [33]. Apparently endogenous nitric oxide produced in the endothelium blocks the vasorelaxing effects of exogenous nitric oxide from nitrate vasodilators; thus endothelial dysfunction increases the vasodilating effects of organic nitrates [32, 35]. Diminished basal endothelial NO formation could be another explanation for the greater efficacy of nitrates on venous vessels.

This special hemodynamic action profile of organic nitrates explains their exceptional anti-ischemic efficacy. Decreased ventricular filling pressure due to reduced preload, direct dilation of stenotic vascular segments, increased compliance of great arteries, and reduced peripheral resistance lead to an improved balance of oxygen requirement and supply. In addition to that nitrates are more or less potent inhibitors of platelet aggregation [20, 21].

Although there is no doubt about the usefulness of organic nitrates in the treatment of ischemic syndromes in coronary heart disease, there are cardiovascular disorders where their efficacy still needs to be assessed. Among these is the use of nitrates in the therapy of heart failure, especially in combination with ACE inhibitors. All major controlled studies concerning the efficacy of organic nitrates in the treatment of chronic heart failure were conducted before ACE inhibitors were available and there are no data about the usefulness of combination therapy of nitrates and ACE inhibitors.

Another area that still needs to be explored is the use of nitrates in the post-myocardial infarction period. Large trials involving more than 80,000 patients have shown that the use of nitrates in the post-myocardial infarction therapy does not improve the patients' prognosis. However, patients with basically normal ventricular function were included in these studies, thus it is questionable if the results can be applied to patients with ventricular dysfunction.

An important limitation of the use of organic nitrates is the development of nitrate tolerance. Clinically, this problem is solved by intermittent application with drug-free periods. There are, however, new approaches that could lead to extended efficacy. We shall have a look at these approaches which could lead to an increased exploitation of the therapeutic potential of organic nitrates in due course.

Role of nitrates in therapy of heart failure

Several theoretical and clinical aspects lead to the assumption of a therapeutic efficacy of nitrates in the therapy of chronic heart failure. The hemodynamic effects, including reduced preload and afterload, decreased left ventricular filling pressure as well as decreased pulmonary hypertension, should relieve symptoms of the disease. Studies by Judgutt et al. [16] involving patients with previous myocardial infarction proved that nitrates are effective in the prevention of ventricular remodeling, which ultimately leads to ventricular enlargement and subsequent heart failure. Recent studies point to a diminished endothelium-dependent vasodilation in heart failure which improved under treatment with nitrate vasodilators [34].

The effects of nitrate therapy on mortality of patients with mild to moderate heart failure was proven for the first time in the V-HeFT-I-Study (Vasodilator Heart Failure Trial) [6]. In this randomized, placebo-controlled study, the usefulness of vasodilator therapy with prazosin or a combination of hydralazine and isosorbide dinitrate (ISDN) was studied on 642 patients already treated with digoxin and diuretics. The combination of hydralazine and ISDN was chosen as pathophysiologic reasoning assumed a balanced reduction of left ventricular preload and afterload. At the end of the average test period of 2.3 years, a significant reduction in mortality was apparent for the combination therapy but not for monotherapy with prazosin. Thus, it had been proven for the first time that isosorbide dinitrate in combination with hydralazine improved the prognosis of patients with heart failure. With the introduction of ACE inhibitors, a study comparing these two efficient therapies seemed appropriate. This comparison was done during the V-HeFT-II-Study [7]. 804 patients with mild to moderate heart failure on a basis regimen of digoxin and diuretics were given either enalapril (20 mg/day) or a combination of hydralazine (300 mg/day) and isosorbide dinitrate (160 mg/day). The study showed that, after 2 years, patients treated with enalapril had a significantly greater reduction in mortality (18 %) compared to patients treated with the combination hydralazine-isosorbide dinitrate (25 %). The ejection fraction (Fig. 1) and the maximum oxygen consumption on exertion increased more in the patients with nitrate therapy. The study showed a greater prognostic effect of the therapy with enalapril, but a better improvement of symptoms following combination therapy with hydralazine and ISDN.

The superior effect of enalapril on mortality in this study as well as the positive effects of ACE inhibitors in subsequent studies [30, 36, 37, 38] established their position in the treatment of heart failure. The combination of hydralazine and isosorbide dinitrate was used as alternative therapy in cases of intolerance to ACE inhibitors. The mechanism of hydralazine action in combination with isosorbide dinitrate has been discussed widely, but it is yet undetermined what part hydralazine plays in the efficacy of the combination. Reduction of afterload alone, such as prazosin showed in the V-HeFT-I-Study, does not reduce mortality. Currently, the hypothesis that hydralazine blocks the development of nitrate tolerance and thus increases the effect of nitrates is widely accepted. There are animal [5] as well as human pharmacological studies [11] supporting this hypothesis. According to recent studies hydralazine inhibits a vascular NADH oxidase which is responsible for increased formation of oxygen radicals in heart failure [29]. These superoxide anions inactivate endogenous and exogenous nitric oxide, thus leading to endothelial dysfunction.

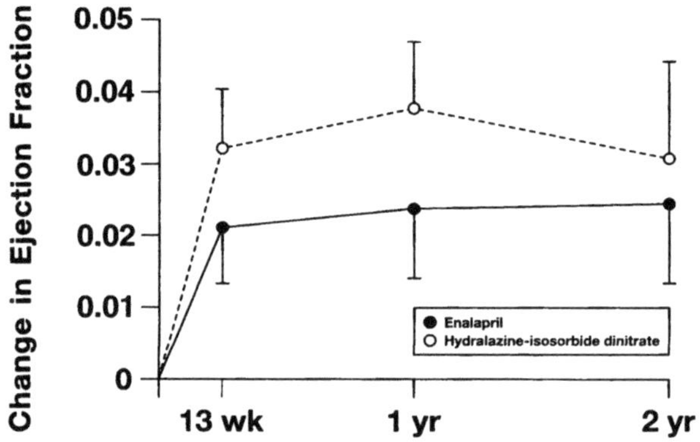

Fig. 1 Change in ejection fraction (confidence interval 95 %) during a therapy of 2 years.
A total of 804 patients with heart failure and already on digoxin and diuretics was additionally treated with either enalapril or hydralazine-isosorbide dinitrate. Compared to the initial value the ejection fraction increased significantly more in patients treated with hydralazine-isosorbide dinitrate than in those treated with enalapril after 13 weeks of treatment ($p < 0.05$). Results of the V-HeFT-II-Study [7].

The proven therapeutic efficacy of ACE inhibitors and nitrates in heart failure therapy leads to the question of a usefulness of a combination of these agents. Surprisingly, there are no studies addressing this question. One reason for this may be that there is no economic incentive for pharmaceutical companies to pay for studies involving substances that are patent-free. Based on theoretical assumptions and clinical experience a combination of ACE inhibitors and nitrate should be useful (Tab. 1). Both groups improve the hemodynamics of patients with heart failure by reducing right and left ventricular pressure, pulmonary hypertension and systemic vascular resistance, and by increasing the stroke volume. Activation of the renin-angiotensin-aldosterone systems by organic nitrates is inhibited through concomitant application of ACE inhibitors. As activation of the renin-angiotensin-aldosterone systems seems to play an important part in the development of nitrate tolerance [17, 19, 26] concurrent treatment with ACE inhibitors can inhibit or diminish tolerance [8, 12, 17, 31]. Although ACE inhibitors do not possess antianginal properties studies have shown that concurrent use of ACE inhibitors increases the antianginal efficacy of ISDN [24] and transdermal nitroglycerin [25]. This could be of special importance for treatment of ischemic heart failure. The V-HeFT-I-Study showed an effect of isosorbide dinitrate-hydralazine on mortality and several large studies proved the same for ACE inhibitors in heart failure patients. This leads to the question whether or not a combination of nitrate and ACE inhibitor could show additive effects. The ACE inhibitor should be better tolerated by most patients than hydralazine, whose usefulness is restricted by a number of specific side-effects such as lupus erythematosus, serum sickness, hemolytic anemia, and glomerulonephritis syndrome.

So far, there are only two smaller studies concerning a combination therapy.

Table 1 Reasons for combination of ACE inhibitors and nitrates in the therapy of heart failure

- Addition of beneficial hemodynamic effects
  - Reduction of: right and left ventricular filling pressure
    - pulmonary artery pressure
    - peripheral vascular resistance
  - Increase of: stroke volume, ejection fraction
- Compensation of nitrate-induced reflex activation of RAA system with ACE inhibitors
- Inhibition or reduction of nitrate tolerance with ACE inhibitors
- Augmentation of anti-ischemic efficacy of nitrates with ACE inhibitors
- Improved prognosis following treatment with both groups
- Better tolerability (compared to a combination of hydralazine and ISDN)

In one study, 10 patients with heart failure and treatment with captopril (10 mg) received additional therapy with either isosorbide dinitrate (40 mg q.i.d.) or placebo for twenty-four hours. Using a right heart catheter the hemodynamic effect of captopril or captopril plus isosorbide dinitrate was assessed [23]. Isosorbide dinitrate improved the preload-reducing efficacy of captopril, which on its own was only moderately effective. It is worth to point out that even after frequent application of isosorbide dinitrate the initial decrease of pulmonary artery pressure remained lowered in patients with ACE inhibitor therapy, a fact that was seen as a sign of diminished tolerance formation.

Recently, the same research group published the first long-term study of therapeutic efficacy of nitrate therapy in patients already treated with ACE inhi-

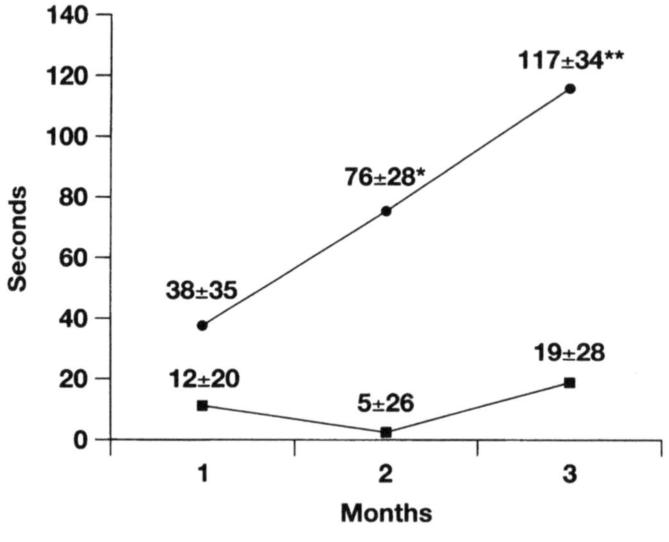

Fig. 2 Change in exercise time on a bicycle ergometer during 3 months of therapy with nitroglycerin (•) or placebo (■). Data from 20 patients with heart failure (NYHA II-III) treated with diuretics, digitalis, and ACE inhibitors who received additional therapy with transdermal nitroglycerin patches (50 to 100 mg/day; 12 hours daily) or placebo in a cross-over study [9]; $* < 0.01$, $**p < 0.03$.

bitors [9]. This study involved 29 patients with heart failure (NYHA class II–III) that were treated intermittently (12 hours daily) with high-dose transdermal nitroglycerin patches (2–4 mg/hr) over three months in a cross-over study. All patients were already treated with captopril (on average 89 mg/day), furosemide, and digoxin. Target measure was treadmill exercise duration. This measure improved continuously over the three month period and the overall increase at the end of the study was approx. 30 % (Fig. 2). On top of that, nitrate therapy showed a significant reduction of both endsystolic and enddiastolic ventricular diameter and a 25 % increase in shortening fraction as a sign of improved systolic myocardial function. The higher rate of symptomatic improvement caused by nitrates in patients already on ACE inhibitors should be due to an improved hemodynamic profile. Anti-ischemic efficacy on its own cannot explain this phenomenon, as only 7 of 29 patients suffered from ischemic heart failure. The positive effect of organic nitrate on improvement of endothelial function of heart failure patients [34] could increase the compliance of arterial vessels, thus increasing the exercise level.

This study showed for the first time that nitrates have a marked additional effect on the symptoms of patients with heart failure who are already on ACE inhibitors. Whether or not this symptomatic improvement also improves the long-term prognosis of patients has to be studied further.

Role of nitrates in the post-myocardial infarction therapy

Whereas there is no doubt about the usefulness of nitroglycerin in acute myocardial infarction, a fact that has been included in the guidelines of the task force of the American College of Cardiology/American Heart Association [1], its use in treatment in the post-infarction period has been questioned by the results of two large randomized studies.

In GISSI-3 [10] 19,394 patients with acute myocardial infarction were randomized within 24 hours of onset of symptoms and either treated with lisinopril (10 mg/day), transdermal nitroglycerin patch (10 mg/day, 14 hrs daily), or a combination therapy of both substances for a period of 6 weeks. The study showed a significant reduction in mortality and combined endpoint (mortality and severe left ventricular dysfunction) for lisinopril treatment, but none for nitroglycerin. However, the reduction in mortality was highest for combination therapy.

The larger ISIS-4 study [13] involved 58,050 patients who again were randomized within 24 hours of onset of symptoms. For the next 4 weeks they were either treated with captopril (50 mg b.d.), isosorbide 5-mononitrate (60 mg daily), or magnesium sulfate (72 mmol for 24 hours). This study showed a significant reduction in mortality for captopril therapy and no change for isosorbide-5-mononitrate therapy, as well. Magnesium therapy seemed to increase mortality after 5 weeks of treatment. The results of these two studies lead to the conclusion that nitrates are not indicated for systematic treatment of patients after myocardial infarction. However, this conclusion has been questioned. One point of criticism is that both trials studied a rather selected group of patients, a point which is supported by the low mortality (approx. 7%) and the high incidence of thrombolytic therapy (approx. 70%). Even more important could be that more than half the patients of the placebo group received intravenous or oral nitrates during the acute stage. Most patients had a normal left ventricular function (only 5% of all patients in GISSI-3 had an ejection fraction of less than 40%). It has been shown that patients with left ventricular dysfunction after myocardial infarction have a progressive ventricular dilatation which is an independent determinant for mortality [41]. On the other hand there are convincing data from animal studies indicating that continuous nitrate therapy reduces ventricular remodeling after infarction, thus leading to an improved ventricular function [14].

A study recently published by Mahmarian et al. [22] looked at the effect of long-term nitrate therapy on ventricular remodeling after myocardial infarction. This multicenter, placebo-controlled, double-blind study involved 291 patients with previous myocardial infarction who were treated with three different doses of transdermal nitroglycerin patches (0.4 mg/hr, 0.8 mg/hr, and 1.6 mg/hr) for six months. During the therapy left ventricular enlargement and function were monitored. The nitroglycerin therapy was intermittent (12 hours daily) and ventricular volume and ejection fraction were measured by gated radionuclide angiography. After six months of therapy with nitroglycerin endsystolic and enddiastolic volume had increased less than in the placebo group. This effect was strongest in the group treated with the lowest nitrate dose (0.4 mg/hr), which even showed a decreased volume compared to the initial volume three days after the myocardial infarction (Fig. 3). Analysis of the different subgroups showed that a reduced ventricular enlargement could only be shown for patients that already had an initially reduced ventricular function (ejection fraction < 40 %). These patients showed a marked increase of the volume index under placebo therapy (approx. 20 ml/m^2), while treatment with 0.4 mg/hr nitroglycerin decreased the index by some 10 ml/m^2 (Fig. 4). After discontinuation of nitrate therapy for one week this effect partially disappeared, but there was still evidence that it was there, although weaker.

The results of this study prove that nitrates have a similar effect on ventricular enlargement as ACE inhibitors [18] and that this effect is primarily limited to patients with reduced ventricular function. Most of the time these are patients with anterior wall myocardial infarction. It does not come as a surprise that nitrate efficacy was most pronounced in patients that had not been treated with ACE inhibitors. Yet, there is some additional effect surpassing ACE inhibitor efficacy. The study shows that our knowledge regarding the thera-

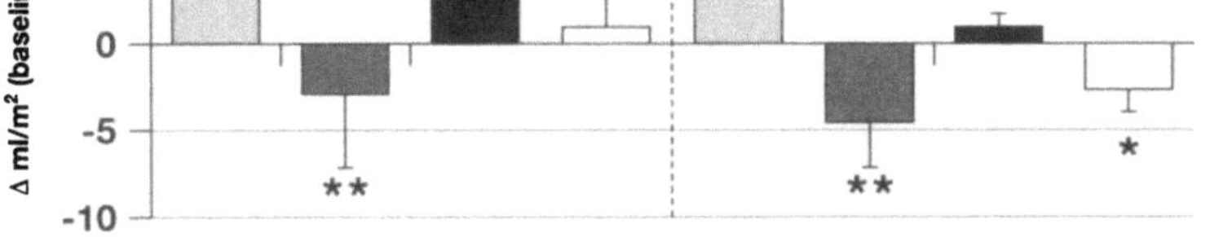

Fig. 3 Change in enddiastolic and endsystolic volume index for 291 patients with myocardial infarction who received either placebo or transdermal nitroglycerin patches (0.4 mg/hr, 0.8 mg/hr, or 1.6 mg/hr) for a period of 6 months starting on the third day after the myocardial infarction. The changes relate to the initial values prior to onset of therapy [22].

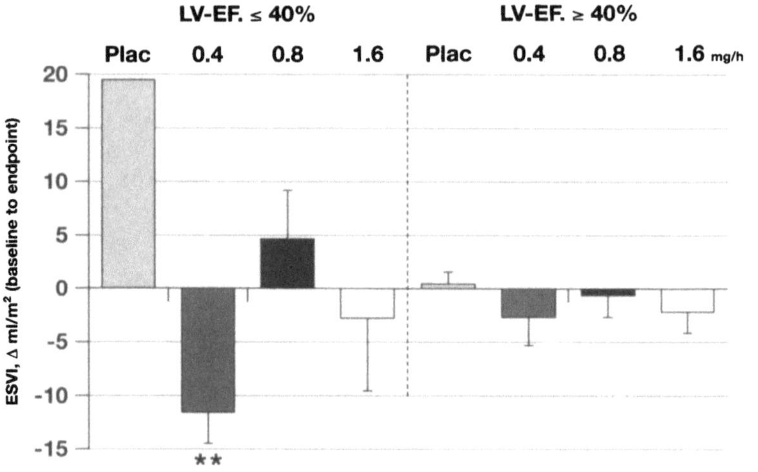

Abb. 4 Change in endsystolic volume index depending on the initial ejection fraction (lower or higher than 40 %); same patients and treatment as in Fig. 3 [22].

peutic usefulness of nitrate in the post-myocardial infarction period is far from being comprehensive and that more studies addressing these problems may lead to an expanded therapeutic use of nitrates.

Nitrate tolerance – strategies for prevention

Development of nitrate tolerance after continuous application is an important limitation of the usefulness of organic nitrates. A nitrate-free period of 12 to 16 hours to sustain the susceptibility of the vascular smooth muscle must be adhered to. A nitrate vasodilator with 24 hour efficacy would be quite a therapeutic achievement. We already discussed that ACE inhibitors have the potential to inhibit tolerance development. However, use of this combination therapy requires in addition an indication for ACE inhibitors. Advanced knowledge concerning the mechanisms of tolerance seems to indicate that it could well be inhibited by concurrent application of hemodynamically inert agents, such as antioxidants. It has been shown that superoxide anions play an important part in the formation of nitrate tolerance [27]. A nitrate-induced activation of the RAA system apparently activates a membrane-bound NADH-dependent oxidase, which in turn produces free oxygen radicals. Nitric oxide is inactivated by these superoxide anions. The forma-tion of superoxide anions could be blocked by inhibition of the RAA system (e.g., by ACE inhibitors, angiotensin receptor blockers) and the inactivation of NO could be prevented by application of antioxidants [28].

Watanabe et al. [40] were able to demonstrate that vitamin E in doses of 200 mg t.i.d. prevented a loss of efficacy (measured as nitrate-induced increased perfusion of the forearm) of transdermal nitroglycerin patches (10 mg/24 hrs) in patients with coronary heart disease and healthy volunteers that was common after three days of treatment. Furthermore, the authors reported that vitamin C can prevent tolerance in patients with heart failure after continuous i.v. infusion of nitroglycerin over 24 hours. The infusion rate was gradually increased until the pulmonary capillary wedge pressure (PCWP) had been reduced by some 30 % and this infusion rate was kept up for 24 hours (Fig. 5). The placebo group showed signs of tolerance development after about 12 hours when the pressure began to rise again, but the group with vitamin C therapy (55 µg/kg/min intravenously) did not show any change in the initially achieved hemodynamic effect. The cGMP level in thrombocytes, measured at the same time, showed the same pattern. In the placebo group it increased with increasing infusion rate of nitroglycerin and started to drop after twelve hours indicating tolerance induction. This drop was prevented by concomitant infusion of vitamin C.

Similar results have been reported by Bassenge et al. [4]. These authors were able to prevent development of hemodynamic nitrate tolerance, which was induced in healthy volunteers by continuous application of a transdermal nitroglycerin patch for 3 days, by concomitant application of vitamin C (500 mg t.i.d.). Vitamin C also prevented typical changes in platelet function (thrombin-induced increase of intracellular calcium concentration and increased thrombin-induced platelet aggregation).

A

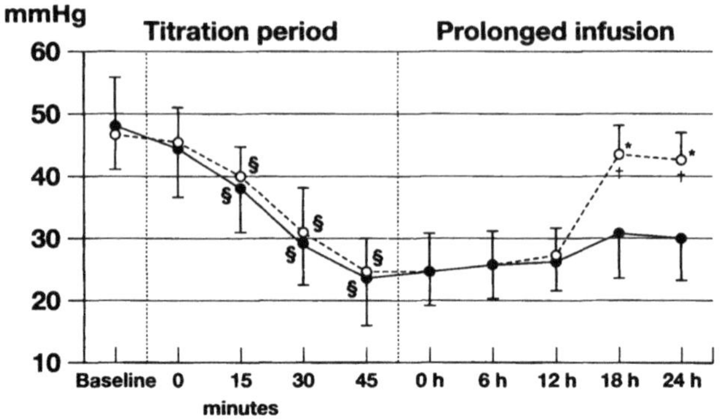

B

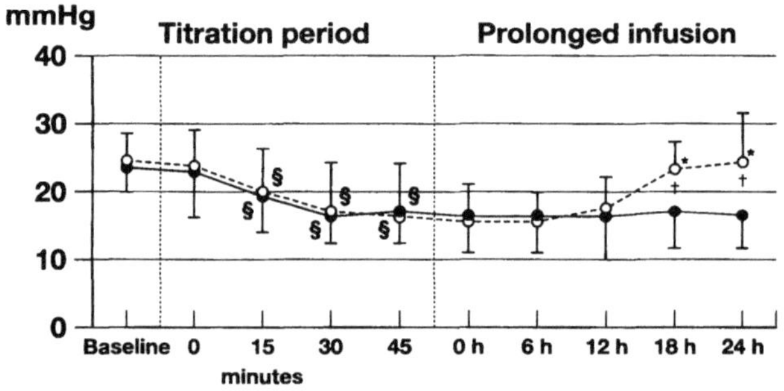

Fig. 5 Change in median pulmonary artery pressure (A) and median pulmonary capillary pressure (B) in patients with heart failure. The patients received i.v. infusion of nitroglycerin until the pulmonary capillary wedge pressure was reduced by 30% (titration period, left side of diagram). This infusion rate was kept constant for the next 24 hours (prolonged infusion, right side of diagram). Patients receiving placebo (o) showed a pressure increase after about twelve hours as nitrate tolerance developed. In patients with vitamin C application (•) the initial reduction in pressure remained constant throughout the 24 hour period [40]; †p < 0.01 vs. vitamin C group; §p < 0.05 vs. minute 0.

These results support the goal of achieving hemodynamic efficacy of nitrate therapy for 24 hours. This would be a major therapeutic innovation and, probably, could open up other indications, e.g., treatment of systolic hypertension in elderly patients.

The fact that organic nitrates are well established drugs which have been used for a long time does not mean that their therapeutic value has been explored comprehensively. New advances in the pathophysiology of diseases and in mechanisms of drug actions could open up new therapeutic options as well as help to improve their usefulness in already established treatment areas.

References

[1] ACC/AHA Task Force Report: Guidelines for the early management of patients with acute myocardial infarction. J. Am. Coll. Cardiol. 16 (1990) 249–292.

[2] Acute Infarction Ramipril Efficacy (AIRE) study investigators: Effect of ramipril on mortality and morbidity of survivors of acute myocardial infarction with clinical evidence of heart failure. Lancet 342 (1993) 821–828.

[3] Bassenge, E., D.J. Stewart: Effects of nitrates in various vascular sections and regions. Z. Kardiol. 75 (1986) 1–7.

[4] Bassenge, E., N. Fink, M. Skatchkov et al.: Dietary supplement with Vitamin C prevents nitrate tolerance. J. Clin. Invest. 102 (1998) 1–5.

[5] Bauer, J.A. and H.-L. Fung: Concurrent hydralazine administration prevents nitroglycerin-induced hemodynamic tolerance in experimental heart failure. Circulation 84 (1991) 35–39.

[6] Cohn, J.N., D.G. Archibald, S. Ziesche et al.: Effect of vasodilator therapy on mortality in chronic congestive heart failure. N. Engl. J. Med. 314 (1986), 1547–1552.

[7] Cohn, J.N., G. Johnson, S. Ziesche et al.: A comparison of enalapril with hydralazine-isosorbide dinitrate in the treatment of chronic congestive heart failure. N. Engl. J. Med. 325 (1991) 303–310.

[8] Cotter, G., E. Metzkor-Cotter, E. Kaluski et al.: Usefulness of Losartan, Captopril and Furosemide in preventing nitrate tolerance and improving control of unstable angina pectoris. Am. J. Cardiol. 82 (1998) 1024–1029.

[9] Elkayam, U., J.V. Johnson, A. Shotan et al.: Double-blind, placebo-controlled study to evaluate the effect of organic nitrates in patients with chronic heart failure treated with angiotensin-converting enzyme inhibition. Circulation 99 (1999) 2652–2657.

[10] GISSI-3 Investigators: Effects of lisinopril and transdermal glyceryl trinitrate singly and together on 6-week mortality and ventricular function after acute myocardial infarction. Lancet 343 (1994) 1115–1122.

[11] Gogia, H., A. Mehra, S. Parikh et al.: Prevention of tolerance to hemodynamic effects of nitrates with concomitant use of hydralazine in patients with chronic heart failure. J. Am. Coll. Cardiol. 26 (1995) 1575–1580.

[12] Heitzer, T., H. Just, C. Brockhoff et al.: Long term nitroglycerin treatment is associated with supersensitivity to vasoconstrictors in men with stable coronary artery disease: prevention by concomitant treatment with captopril. J. Am. Cardiol. 31 (1998) 83–88.

[13] ISIS-4: A randomized factorial trial assessing early oral captopril, oral mononitrate, and intravenous magnesium sulphate in 58.050 patients with suspected acute myocardial infarction. Lancet 345 (1995) 669–685.

[14] Jugdutt, B.I., M.I Kahn: Effect of prolonged nitrate therapy on left ventricular remodeling after canine acute myocardial infarction. Circulation 89 (1994) 2297–2307.

[15] Jugdutt, B.I., M.I. Khan, G.E. Blinston: Impact of left ventricular unloading after late reperfusion of canine anterior myocardial infarction on remodeling and function using isosorbide-5-mononitrate. Circulation 92 (1995) 926–934.

[16] Jugdutt, B.I.: Effects of nitrate therapy on ventricular remodeling and function. Am. J. Cardiol. 72(suppl) (1993) 161G–168G.

[17] Katz, R.J., W.S. Levy, L. Buff et al.: Prevention of nitrate tolerance with angiotensin converting enzyme inhibitors. Circulation 83 (1991) 1271–1277.

[18] Konstam, M.A., M.F. Rousseau, M.W. Kronenberg et al.: Effects of the angiotensin converting enzyme inhibitor enalapril on the long-term progression of left ventricular dysfunction in patients with heart failure. Circulation 86 (1992) 431–438.

[19] Kurz, S., U. Hink, G.Nickenig et al.: Evidence for a causal role of the renin-angiotensin system in nitrate tolerance. Circulation 99 (1999) 3181–3187.

[20] Lam, J.Y.T., J.H. Chesebro, V. Fuster: Platelets, vasoconstriction and nitroglycerin during arterial wall injury: A new antithrombotic role for an old drug. Circulation 78 (1988) 712–716.

[21] Loscalzo, J.: Antiplatelet and antithrombotic effects of organic nitrates. Am. J. Cardiol. 70 (1992) 18B–22B.

[22] Mahmarian, J.J., L.A. Moyé, D. A. Chinoy, et al.: Transdermal nitroglycerin patch therapy improves left ventricular function and prevents remodeling after acute myocardial infarction. Circulation 97 (1998) 2017–2024.

[23] Mehra, A., E. Ostrzega, A. Shotan et al.: Persistent hemodynamic improvement with short-term nitrate therapy in patients with chronic congestive heart failure already treated with captopril. Am. J. Cardiol. 70 (1992) 1310–1314.

[24] Metelitsa, V., S.Y. Martsevoch, M.P. Kozyreva et al.: Non-SH containing ACE inhibitors perindopril potentiates the efficacy of isosorbide dinitrate in patients with stable angina pectoris. Eur. Heart J. 12 (1991) 81.
[25] Muiesan, M.L., E. Boni, M. Castellano et al.: Effects of transdermal nitroglycerin in combination with an ACE inhibitor in patients with chronic stable angina pectoris. Eur. Heart J. 14 (1993) 1701–1708
[26] Münzel, T., E. Bassenge: Long-term angiotensin-converting enzyme inhibition with high dose enalapril retards nitrate tolerance in large epicardial arteries and prevents rebound coronary vasoconstriction in vivo. Circulation 93 (1996) 2052–2058.
[27] Münzel, T., H. Sayegh, B.A. Freeman, et al.: Evidence for enhanced vascular superoxide anion production in nitrate tolerance: a novel mechanism of tolerance and cross tolerance. J. Clin. Invest. 95 (1995) 187–194.
[28] Münzel, T., S. Kurz, T, Heitzer, et al.: New insights into mechanism underlying nitrate tolerance. Am. J. Cardiol. 77 (1996) 24C–30C.
[29] Münzel, T., S. Kurz, M. Tarpey et al.: Hydralazin prevents nitroglycerin tolerance by inhibiting activation of a membrane-bound NADH oxidase; a new action for an old drug. J. Clin. Invest. 98 (1996) 1465–1470.
[30] Pfeffer, M.A., E. Braunwald, L.A: Moye et al. on behalf of the SAVE investigators: Effect of captopril on mortality and morbidity in patients with left ventricular dysfunction after myocardial infarction: Results of the Survival and Ventricular Enlargement trial. N. Eng. J. Med. 327 (1992) 669–677.
[31] Pizulli, L., A. Hagendorff, M. Zirbes et al.: Influence of captopril on nitroglycerin mediated vasodilatation and development of nitrate tolerance in arterial and venous circulation. Am. Heart J. 131 (1996) 343–349.
[32] Pohl, U., R. Busse: Endothelium-derived relaxant factor inhibits effects of nitrocompounds in isolated arteries. Am. J. Physiol. 252 (1987) H307–H313.
[33] Rafflenbeul, W., E. Bassenge, P. Lichtlen: Competition between endothelium-dependent and nitroglycerin-induced coronary vasodilation (Konkurrenz zwischen endothelabhängiger und Nitroglycerin-induzierter koronarer Vasodilation) Z. Kardiol. 78 (1989) 45–57.
[34] Schwarz, M., S.D. Katz, L. Demopoulos et al.: Enhancement of endothelium-dependent vasodilation by low-dose nitroglycerin in patients with congestive heart failure. Circulation 89 (1994) 1609–1614.
[35] Shirasaki, T., C. Su, T.J.-F. Lee et al.: Endothelial modulation of vascular relaxation to nitrovasodilators in ageing and hypertension. J. Pharmacol. Exp. Ther. 239 (1986) 861–866.
[36] The Acute Infarction Ramipril Efficacy (Aire) Study investigators: Effects of Ramipril on mortality of survivors of acute myocardial infarction with clinical evidence of heart failure. Lancet 342 (1993) 821–828.

[37] The Consensus Trial Study Group: Effects of enalapril on mortality in severe congestive heart failure: Results of the Cooperative North Scandinavian Enalapril Survival Study (CONSENSUS). N. Eng. J. Med. 316 (1987) 1429–1436.

[38] The SOLVD investigators: Effect of Enalapril on survival in patients with reduced left ventricular ejection fraction and congestive heart failure. N. Eng. J. Med. 325 (1991) 293–302.

[39] Watanabe, H., M. Kakihana, S. Ohtsuka et al.: Randomized, double-blind, placebo-controlled study of supplemental vitamin E on attenuation of the development of nitrate tolerance. Circulation 96 (1997) 2545–2550.

[40] Watanabe, H., M. Kakihana, S. Ohtsuka et al.: Randomized, double-blind, placebo-controlled study of ascorbate on the preventive effect of nitrate tolerance in patients with congestive heart failure. Circulation 97 (1998) 886–891.

[41] White, H.D., R.M. Norris, M.A. Brown, et al.: Left ventricular end-systolic volume as the major determinant of survival after recovery from myocardial infarction. Circulation 76 (1987) 44–51.

Overview of nitrate therapy

J. O. Parker

Organic nitrates are extensively used in the management of coronary artery disease. They are given not only to patients with stable angina pectoris, but also to those with unstable angina, acute myocardial infarction and heart failure. This overview will relate primarily to the use of organic nitrates in patients with chronic, stable angina pectoris, but many of the principles enunciated are relevant to the other clinical situations.

Pharmacology of organic nitrates

Commonly used organic nitrates include nitroglycerin (glyceryl trinitrate), isosorbide dinitrate, and isosorbide mononitrate. Although not commonly prescribed in North America, erythrityl tetranitrate and pentaerythrityl tetranitrate are used extensively in many parts of the world. The nitrates are rapidly absorbed from the gastrointestinal tract, skin and mucous membranes. When given orally, isosorbide dinitrate and nitroglycerin undergo extensive first pass hepatic metabolism [4]. The plasma half-life of nitroglycerin is approximately three minutes, while the active metabolites of nitroglycerin (1–2 glyceryl dinitrate and 1–3 glyceryl dinitrate) are biologically active and have half-lives of 30–40 minutes [1, 4].

Isosorbide dinitrate has significant hemodynamic and antianginal effects, but it is rapidly metabolized, since it has a plasma half-life of approximately 40 minutes. Its major metabolites, isosorbide-2-mononitrate and isosorbide-5-mononitrate, are biologically active and their half-lives are approximately

2 and 4 hours respectively [4]. Isosorbide-5-mononitrate is completely bioavailable and does not undergo first pass hepatic metabolism. The prolonged effects of isosorbide dinitrate are related primarily to the mononitrate metabolites.

Mechanism of action of the organic nitrates

The organic nitrates are pro-drugs and must be biodegraded to have therapeutic effects. This involves denitration with the formation of nitric oxide. Nitric oxide activates quanylyl cyclase leading to the conversion of guanosine triphosphate to cycle guanosine monophosphate which, in turn, causes vasodilation by reducing the availability of calcium to the contractile proteins in vascular smooth muscle [5, 9, 15]. How the nitrates undergo denitration and how nitric oxide is released is still unclear. At one time, it was felt that reduced sulfhydryl groups were an essential substrate for bioconversion [20], but they are probably only required as a co-factor.

Nitric oxide is identical to the endothelium-derived relaxing factor. Nitric oxide, in addition to its vasodilating properties, reduces platelet adhesion and aggregation and these effects have been shown to be provided by the nitrates [17]. Nitric oxide is also involved in the control of endothelial function, vascular growth, and myocardium contractility [16]. Endothelial dysfunction is associated with diminished nitric oxide production and it is possible that the organic nitrates, by providing nitric oxide, might be beneficial in such conditions. This hypothesis is attractive, but has not been tested in humans as of yet.

Nitrates cause vasodilatation in both the venous and arterial systems. The nitrates dilate capacitance veins and thus lower venous return, left ventricular volume and filling pressures, changes that reduce left ventricular preload. In the doses used clinically, the nitrates have no effect on the arteriolar resistance vessels but dilate conductive arteries. This results in diminished impedance and, in combination with reduced left ventricular volume, lowers afterload. These effects reduce myocardial oxygen requirements. The nitrates dilate epicardial coronary arteries including stenotic segments, particularly those with eccentric lesions and also dilate intracoronary collateral vessels. These changes increase blood flow and improve its distribution to ischemic areas. The reduction of left ventricular filling pressures, regularly seen with nitrates, also improves subendocardial blood flow. These multiple nitrate effects thus improve the mismatch between myocardial oxygen demand and supply that characterize the ischemic syndromes in patients with coronary artery disease.

Nitroglycerin in the treatment of anginal attacks

Nitroglycerin is the drug most frequently used for treatment of anginal attacks. This can be given as a sublingual tablet or spray. The spray is desirable in that the sublingual tablets deteriorate once exposed to air, and should be replaced every three months while the spray is stable for at least three years. Isosorbide dinitrate is also available as a sublingual tablet, but is slower in its onset of action.

Nitroglycerin in angina prophylaxis

Sublingual nitroglycerin, tablet or spray

These preparations are very effective in the prophylactic treatment of angina [31]. Patients with predictable angina may prevent symptoms by taking nitroglycerin two or three minutes prior to activities and this approach often does away with the need for other antianginal therapy.

Oral nitroglycerin

Nitroglycerin is available in sustained release preparations and is marketed to be given every 8–12 hours. This dosing regimen increases exercise tolerance for up to four hours after the morning dose, but there are no data demonstrating efficacy throughout the dosing interval [40]. The infrequent development of headaches suggest that there may be low bioavailability of these products, or such extensive hepatic metabolism that they exert little systemic effects. Without firm data, however, one would be hesitant to recommend the use of the sustained release preparations of nitroglycerin.

Transdermal nitroglycerin

Nitroglycerin ointment has been employed for many years and has clinically important anginal effects [14]. There are, however, limited data relating to long-term therapy with this preparation. With the evidence that transdermal nitroglycerin patches are effective if given intermittently, one would expect that nitroglycerin ointment, if given in adequate doses and providing a 12-hour nitrate-free period is maintained, that this would be effective in anti-anginal prophylaxis.

Nitroglycerin transdermal patches

Transdermal nitroglycerin patches were originally approved to be applied once daily and left in place for 24 hours. There were, however, no clinical trials documenting the efficacy of this regime when these preparations were approved by the Food and Drug Administration in the United States. Subsequent small studies provided variable results regarding their efficacy, but the majority of studies indicated that tolerance occurred when this regime was employed [25, 32]. A large study carried out in the United States with 562 patients with continuous nitroglycerin transdermal patch application documented that tolerance developed within 24 hours. Tolerance could not be overcome by increasing doses up to 4.2 mg/hr [34]. The provision of a patch-free period is effective in preventing, or at least reducing, tolerance. Studies have documented that a regime of 12 hours on, 12 hours off is effective in improving exercise tolerance in patients with chronic, stable angina pectoris [7, 30].

Isosorbide dinitrate in angina prophylaxis

Sublingual isosorbide dinitrate

Sublingual isosorbide dinitrate is useful in the prevention of angina. It has a longer half-life than nitroglycerin and can provide prophylactic effects for up to an hour [12].

Standard formulation isosorbide dinitrate

Standard formulation isosorbide dinitrate is rapidly absorbed and provides antianginal effects for up to eight hours when initially given. However, during long-term therapy given four times daily, with the last done given at bedtime, partial tolerance to the hemodynamic and antianginal effects develops [37]. Tolerance develops despite higher plasma concentrations during the sustained phase than was seen with the original dose. Later studies, in which isosorbide dinitrate was given three times daily with a tablet-free period of 14 hours, tolerance did not develop [27]. This study assessed the antianginal effects after the morning dose only and there are limited data relating to the effects after the second and third dose of isosorbide dinitrate in this eccentric dosing regimen.

Sustained release isosorbide dinitrate

A variety of sustained release preparations of isosorbide dinitrate are available. Studies have documented that when, given twice daily, 12 hours apart, tolerance develops [33]. When given once daily or in an eccentric fashion with a 12-hour-tablet-free period, tolerance is avoided. The sustained release preparations of isosorbide dinitrate utilized in America are marketed for twice daily administration in doses of 20–80 mg, but there are no data from controlled clinical trials documenting efficacy.

Angina prophylaxis with isosorbide mononitrate

Standard formulation isosorbide-5-mononitrate

Clinical studies have documented that isosorbide mononitrate in standard formulation in doses of 20–40 mg, induce tolerance when given every 12 hours. If, however, these are given in eccentric fashion, that is, twice daily with seven hours between doses, the antianginal effects last for 12 hours [29, 37–39].

Sustained release isosorbide mononitrate

Sustained release preparations of isosorbide mononitrate are available that provide therapeutic plasma drug concentrations for up to 12 hours each day and low concentrations during the latter part of the 24 hour period. A recent multicentre trial has shown that the sustained release therapy in larger doses (120–140 mg) was effective after 12 hours each day during sustained treatment [6].

Nitrates as initial prophylactic therapy

The proven effectiveness of the nitrates in patients with stable angina and their excellent safety profile makes them an effective choice for initial therapy. This is particularly so if patients respond well to short-acting nitroglycerin. The nitrates are also a good choice for initial therapy in patients with angina who have left ventricular dysfunction or mitral regurgitation. Patients who are hypertensive or who have had a previous myocardial infarction, should probably be treated initially with beta blockers. There are no data to suggest that the nitrates are superior to beta adrenergic antagonists or calcium channel antagonists, but nitrates are appropriate initial therapy for many patients with angina pectoris.

Of the current nitrate preparations, only a limited number have been shown to have antianginal and anti-ischemic efficacy for up to 12 hours each day. This includes transdermal nitroglycerin patches, standard formulation isosorbide mononitrate given eccentrically, and controlled release isosorbide dinitrate, given twice daily, eight hours apart.

Combination therapy

The nitrates are commonly prescribed in combination with other antianginal agents if angina is poorly controlled or occurs during the nitrate-free period.

There is little evidence that combination therapy is of greater benefit than monotherapy in the treatment of exertional symptoms. The results of small studies assessing the efficacy of combined therapy with nitrates and beta adrenergic antagonists have been contradictory [2]. Several large trials, assessing the efficacy of oral and transdermal nitrates permitted concurrent therapy with a beta adrenergic antagonist. The nitrates did provide additive effects to the background therapy of beta adrenergic antagonists [6, 29, 30, 36]. It is important to point out, however, that no attempt was made to maximize therapy with the latter agent prior to the administration of the nitrate. There is even less evidence regarding efficacy of triple therapy as is commonly employed in clinical practice [3, 18].

Unstable angina pectoris

Unstable angina pectoris is extremely common and presents particular problems to the cardiologist. Aspirin and heparin are first-line therapies for this condition, and intravenous nitroglycerin is commonly employed. It is in this situation that the problem of nitrate tolerance becomes a difficult one. It is usually necessary to give increasing doses of intravenous nitroglycerin to control symptoms, and rebound ischemia may occur after the discontinuation of intravenous nitroglycerin. These rebound phenomena can be minimized by careful down-titration of nitroglycerin and by the judicious use of oral or transdermal nitrates, beta adrenergic antagonists, or calcium channel blockers during this down-titration phase. During the change from intravenous to oral or transdermal nitroglycerin therapy, it is inappropriate to use intermittent therapy and it may be necessary to utilize incremental dosing during this unstable state.

Nitrate therapy in acute myocardial infarction

The use of the organic nitrates in acute myocardial infarction has shown, in some studies, to reduce infarct size, to prevent infarct expansion, and to reduce left ventricular remodeling. While many of these studies have been relatively small, meta-analyses have shown that intravenous nitroglycerin leads to a 20% reduction in mortality [41]. Recent megatrials, including the ISIS-4, which employed sustained release IS-5-MN [14], and GISSI-3, which employed transdermal nitroglycerin patches [10], showed no effect on 30 day mortality. In these studies, many patients not randomized to receive nitrates, were given these preparations and thus, it is difficult to determine whether or not the administration of nitrates will modify mortality in the early phases of acute myocardial infarction.

Congestive heart failure

The organic nitrates, in intravenous form, are commonly employed in acute congestive heart failure. These agents certainly have a favourable hemodynamic profile in patients with heart failure with reduced preload, afterload, and they may increase ejection fraction, as well as cardiac output. Nitrates also may reduce mitral regurgitation commonly associated with heart failure. The problem of nitrate tolerance is of concern as tolerance develops within a few hours of nitrate administration when patients may still have very significant hemodynamic abnormalities.

In the veterans' administration study, the combination of isosorbide dinitrate and hydralazine given four times daily was shown to reduce mortality in patients with chronic congestive heart failure. This regimen was compared with enalapril in a second study. Those treated with enalapril showed a greater effect on mortality than the nitrate hydralazine group, although exercise tolerance was more improved in patients receiving nitrates and hydralazine. The oral administration of isosorbide dinitrate in chronic congestive heart failure has been extensively reviewed and these investigators have documented diminished hemodynamic effects on left ventricular filling pressures after repeated doses of oral isosorbide dinitrate while intermittent dosing has been more effective. Importantly, it has been demonstrated that the administration of hydralazine has prevented the tolerance associated with frequent oral doses of isosorbide dinitrate [11].

It is clear that the nitrates have important effects that are beneficial in the management of patients with stable angina pectoris, unstable angina pectoris, acute myocardial infarction, and congestive heart failure. The development of tolerance clearly has a negative impact on their effectiveness. If the problem of tolerance could be overcome, then these agents would be even more useful in these clinical situations. At the present time the understanding of the mechanism of tolerance is incomplete. The major hypotheses include (1) sulfhydryl group depletion, (2) neurohormonal activation, (3) plasma volume expansion, and (4) super oxide anion production. It is currently felt that sulfhydryl group depletion is not responsible for tolerance [8]. Neurohormonal activation does occur, but this is not a consistent phenomenon [23, 26, 28]. Plasma volume expansion, by increasing preload, may be related to nitrate tolerance, but diuretic therapy has had variable effects on this response to nitrate therapy [19, 24, 35]. The current hypothesis that is widely accepted is that nitrate therapy leads to the local production of angiotensin II and endothelin I. Oxidative stress leads to increased degradation of nitric oxide, and induces increased sensitivity to vasoconstricting agents [22, 23]. Some animal studies have shown that angiotensin converting enzymes can prevent tolerance but a study in humans showed no such effect [23].

The hypothesis that such oxidative stress is responsible for nitrate tolerance has been tested by the administration of antioxidants. Some studies in animals and man have documented that antioxidant vitamins are associated with diminished nitrate tolerance, but more studies are needed to determine whether antioxidants play a significant role in the prevention of tolerance.

Conclusion

The organic nitrates are effective agents in the management of all phases of patients with coronary artery disease including stable and unstable angina, acute myocardial infarction, and acute and chronic congestive failure. Their clinical efficacy is, however, diminished by the development of tolerance and intermittent or eccentric dosing is required to prevent this phenomenon. To date, there is conflicting evidence regarding the efficacy of adjuvant therapy in the prevention of nitrate tolerance. Thus, at the present time, nitrates should be administered intermittently or eccentrically to provide clinically significant effects for up to 12 hours each day.

References

[1] Armstrong, P.W., J.A. Moffat, G.S. Marks: Arterial-venous nitroglycerin gradient during intravenous infusion in man. Circulation 66 (1982) 1273–1976.

[2] Battock, D.J., H. Alvarez, C.A. Chidsey: Effects of propranolol and isosorbide dinitrate on exercise performance and adrenergic activity in patients with angina pectoris. Circulation 39 (1969) 157–169.

[3] Boden, W., E. Bough, M. Richman et al.: Beneficial effects of high-dose diltiazem in patients with persistent angina on β-blockers and nitrates: a randomized, double-blind, placebo-controlled, cross-over study. Circulation 71 (1985) 1197–1205.

[4] Bogaert, M.G.: Pharmacokinetics of organic nitrates in man: an overview. Eur. Heart J. 9 (1988) 33–37.

[5] Brown, G., E. Bolson, R.B. Peterson et al.: The mechanisms of nitroglycerin action. Stenosis vasodilation as a major component of drug response. Circulation 64 (1981) 1089–1097.

[6] Chrysant, S.G., S.P. Glasser, N. Bittar et al.: Efficacy and safety of extended-release isosorbide mononitrate for stable effort angina pectoris. Am. J. Cardiol. 72 (1993) 1249–1256.

[7] DeMots, H., S.P. Glasser: Intermittent transdermal nitroglycerin therapy in the treatment of chronic stable angina. J. Am. Coll. Card. 13 (1989) 786–788.

[8] Dupuis, J., G. Lalonde, R. Lemieux et al.: Tolerance to intravenous nitroglycerin in patients with congestive heart failure: role of increased intravascular volume, neurohumoral activation and lack of prevention with N-acetylcysteine. J. Am. Coll. Cardiol. 16 (1990) 923–931.

[9] Fung, H.L., S.J. Chung, J.A. Bauer et al.: Biochemical mechanism of organic nitrate action. Am. J. Cardiol. 70 (1992) 4B–10B.

[10] GISSI-3: Effects of lisinopril and transdermal glyceryl trinitrate singly and together on 6 week mortality and ventricular function after acute myocardial infarction. Gruppo Italiano per lo Studio della Sopravivenza nellinfarcto Miocardica. Lancet 343 (1994) 1115–1122.

[11] Gogia, H., A. Mehra, S. Parikh et al.: Prevention of tolerance to hemodynamic effects of nitrates with concomitant use of hydralazine in patients with chronic heart failure. J. Am. Coll. Cardiol. 26 (1995) 1575–1580.

[12] Goldstein, R.S., D.R. Rosing, D.R. Redwood et al.: Clinical and circulatory effects of isosorbide dinitrate: comparison with nitroglycerin. Circulation 43 (1971) 629–634.

[13] ISIS-4: A randomized factorial trial assessing early oral captopril, oral mononitrate, and intravenous magnesium sulphate in 58,050 patients with suspected acute myocardial infarction. ISIS-4 (Fourth International Study of Infarct Survival) Collaborative Group. Lancet 345 (1995) 669–685.

[14] Kala, R., P. Hiroven, A. Gordin et al.: Nitroglycerin ointment is effective for seven hours in severe angina pectoris. Acta Med. Scand. 213 (1983) 165–170.

[15] Katsuki, S., F. Murad: Regulation of adenosine cyclic 3',5'-monophosphate and guanosine cyclic 3',5'-monophosphate and contractility in bovine tracheal smooth muscle. Mol. Pharmacol. 13 (1977) 330–341.

[16] Kelly, R.A., J.L. Balligand, T.W. Smith: Nitric oxide and cardiac function. Circ. Res. 79 (1996) 363–380.

[17] Loscalzo, J: N-Acetylcysteine potentiates inhibition of platelet aggregation by nitroglycerin. J. Clin. Invest. 76 (1985) 703–708.

[18] Meluzin, J., K. Zeman, F. Stetka et al.: Effects of nifedipine and diltiazem on myocardial ischemia in patients with severe stable angina pectoris treated with nitrates and beta blockers. J. Cardiovasc. Pharmacol. 20 (1992) 864–869.

[19] Mohanty, N., A. Wasserman, P. Walker et al.: Prevention of nitroglycerin tolerance with diuretics. Am. Heart J. 130 (1995) 522–527.

[20] Needleman, P., E.M. Johnson: Sulfhydryl requirements for relaxation of vascular smooth muscle. J. Pharmacol. Exp. Ther. 187 (1973) 324–331.

[21] Munzel, T., H. Sayegh, B.A. Freeman et al.: Evidence for enhanced vascular superoxide anion production in nitrate tolerance: a novel mechanism underlying tolerance and cross-tolerance. J. Clin. Invest. 95 (1995) 187–194.

[22] Munzel, T., A. Giaid, S. Kurz et al.: Evidence for a role of endothelin I and protein kinase C in nitroglycerin tolerance. Proc. Natl. Acad. Sci. U.S.A. 92 (1995) 5244–5248.

[23] Parker, J.D., J.O. Parker: Effect of therapy with an angiotensin-converting enzyme inhibitor on hemodynamic and counterregulatory responses during continuous therapy with nitroglycerin. J. Am. Coll. Cardiol. 21 (1993) 1445–1453.

[24] Parker, J.D., A.B. Parker, B. Farrell et al.: The effects of diuretic therapy on the development of tolerance to nitroglycerin and exercise capacity in patients with chronic stable angina. Circulation 93 (1996) 691–696.

[25] Parker, J.O., H.-L. Fung: Transdermal nitroglycerin in angina pectoris. Am. J. Cardiol. 54 (1984) 471–476.

[26] Parker, J.D., B. Farrell, T. Fenton et al.: Counter-regulatory responses to continuous and intermittent therapy with nitroglycerin. Circulation 84 (1991) 2336–2345.

[27] Parker, J., B. Farrell, K. Lahey et al.: Effect of intervals between doses on the development of tolerance to isosorbide dinitrate. N. Engl. J. Med. 316 (1987) 1440–1444.

[28] Parker, J.O., J.D. Parker: Neurohormonal activation during nitrate therapy: a possible mechanism for tolerance. Am. J. Cardiol. 70 (1992) 93B–97B.

[29] Parker, J.O.: Eccentric dosing with isosorbide-5-mononitrate in angina pectoris. Am. J. Cardiol. 72 (1993) 871–786.

[30] Parker, J.O., M.H. Amies, R.W. Hawkinson et al.: Intermittent transdermal nitroglycerin therapy in angina pectoris. Clinically effective without tolerance or rebound. Minitran Efficacy Study Group. Circulation 91 (1995) 1368–1374.

[31] Reichek, N., C. Priest, T. Chandler et al.: Comparison of time of onset of hemodynamic effects of sustained-release buccal nitroglycerin and sublingual nitroglycerin. In: Goldberg, A.A.J., D.G. Parkson (eds.): Modern concepts of nitrate delivery systems. 143–149, London: Royal Society of Medicine, Academic Press: New York, Grune and Stratton, 1983.

[32] Reichek, N., C. Priest, D. Zimrin et al.: Antianginal effects of nitroglycerin patches. Am. J. Cardiol. 54 (1987) 1–7.

[33] Silber, S., A.C. Vogler, K.H. Krause et al.: Induction and circumvention of nitrate tolerance applying different dosage intervals. Am. J. Med. 83 (1987) 860–870.

[34] Steering Committee Transdermal Cooperative Study: Acute and chronic antianginal efficacy of continuous twenty-four application of transdermal nitroglycerin. Am. J. Cardiol. 68 (1992) 1263–1273.

[35] Sussex, B.A., N.R.C. Campbell, M.K. Raju et al.: The antianginal efficacy of isosorbide dinitrate is maintained during diuretic treatment. Clin. Pharmacol. Ther. 56 (1994) 229–234.

[36] Svendsen, J.H., O. Amtorp: Mononitrates in combination with beta blocker therapy in the treatment of severe angina pectoris. Drugs 33 Suppl 4 (1987) 122–124.

[37] Thadani, U., H.-L. Fung, A.C. Darke et al.: Oral isosorbide dinitrate in angina pectoris: Comparison of duration of action and dose response relation during acute and sustained therapy. Am. J. Cardiol. 89 (1982) 1074–1080.

[38] Thadani, U., R. Prasad, S.F. Hamilton et al.: Usefulness of twice-daily isosorbide-5-mononitrate in preventing development of tolerance in angina pectoris. Am. J. Cardiol. 60 (1987) 477–482.

[39] Thadani, U., C.R. Maranda, E. Amsterdam et al.: Lack of pharmacologic tolerance and rebound angina pectoris during twice-daily therapy with isosorbide-5-mononitrate. Ann. Intern. Med. 120 (1994) 353–359.

[40] Winsor, T., H. Berger: Oral nitroglycerin as a prophylactic antianginal drug: clinical, physiologic, and statistical evidence of efficacy based on a three-phase experimental design. Am. Heart J. 90 (1975) 611–626.

[41] Yusef, S., R. Collins, S. MacMahon et al.: Effect of intravenous nitrates on mortality in acute myocardial infarction: an overview of the randomised trials. Lancet 85 (1994) 1088–1092.

Physical exercise of patients with coronary heart disease: effects and importance of nitrates

I. Kruck and G. Kruck

Introduction

It has been known that physical exercise can increase the acute risk of myocardial infarction in patients with coronary heart disease. Extended or sudden physical stress is the trigger in the majority of patients [19]. Emotional stress, heavy meals or hasty eating, cold, or lack of oxygen are causes seen less often.

The so-called TRIMM study, a combined effort of groups in Berlin and Augsburg, took a more detailed look at trigger mechanisms. It showed that the risk of having a myocardial infarction is lower when the subject is at rest, asleep, or engaging in moderate exercise than during heavy work. A subanalysis showed that patients exercising less than four times a week were most likely to have a MI (Fig. 1). Strenuous physical activity doubled the risk, whereas other unusual life events were equally common in the patient and control groups [37]. Similar results were reported by Mittleman, whose study included 1,300 patients with myocardial infarction. The relative risk of experiencing a myocardial infarction was six times higher for the sedentary group than for the group with little physical exercise. A regular exercise schedule of five times or more per week resulted in a relative risk of only 2.4. Thus, patients not participating in any physical exercise are particularly at risk during "acute" strenuous physical stress [23].

In this paper we will attempt to answer the following questions:

- What conclusions can be drawn from studies on primary and secondary prevention through physical exercise?

- What recommendations do we have for patients based on these results?
- How important are nitrates, alone or in combination with other substances, in the cardiac rehabilitation of coronary heart disease patients?
- What is the importance of nitrates in that context, alone or im combination with other drugs?
- What methods are appropriate for determining the stress limit for exercise therapy and assessing therapeutic efficacy?

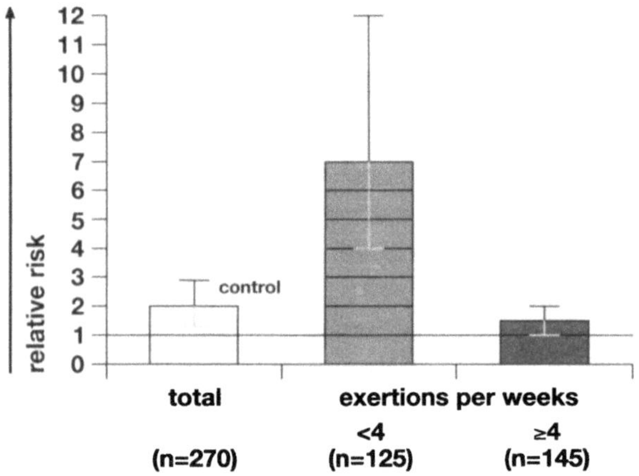

Fig. 1 Relative risk of physical activity within one hour before onset of myocardial infarction (control: relative risk = 1). Patients with physical exertion less than four times per week have a relative risk of 6.9 compared with 1.3 for patients with more than four exertions per week [37].

Exercise as a means of primary prevention

Studies from the 1980s involving large number of patients showed that regular physical exercise can have a positive influence on cardiovascular morbidity and mortality. A study by Morris in 1980 showed that older men (aged 55 to 65) benefited most. The participating 17,944 participating men were asked to engage in heavy physical activity during their leisure time, with a target energy consumption of 7.5 kcal/min. Patients with arterial hypertension and adiposity were included in the study, as well as smokers and those with a family history of coronary heart disease [24].

In a study by Paffenbarger, the age-adjusted cardiovascular mortality for physically active patients was approx. 60 % lower than for the less active control group [29]. A change in lifestyle, even at an advanced age, improved the outlook. In a large study involving 25,000 men and 7,000 women, Blair was able to show that this applies for women, too. The average follow-up period was 7.5 years for women and 8.4 years for men. The study was designed to look for a correlation between cardiorespiratory fitness and cardiovascular mortality while taking the usual risk factors into consideration. Cardiorespiratory fitness was examined using maximal treadmill test. In general, a low level of physical fitness was revealed to be an important predicting factor for cardiovascular mortality. A moderate or very good level of physical fitness reduced the risk of dying from a cardiovascular event considerably. The relative risk of cardiovascular mortality was 1.5 for men, and 2.2 for women, with low physical fitness, i.e., significantly higher than for patients with high fitness levels (Figs. 2 a+b). For men, risk factors such as smoking, high cholesterol level or high blood pressure were other independent predictors. A small, five-month intervention study on the primary prevention of coronary heart disease carried out in Hamburg also showed a reduction in risk factors, as well as an increase in capacity and duration [18]. In 1983 Blair conducted a study involving 750 middle-aged men without known coronary heart disease. He was able to show that regular physical exercise leads to a lower risk for cardiovascular events, while at the same time increasing stress endurance and decreasing risk factors [2, 3].

Exercise as a means of secondary prevention

The NEHDP study (National-Exercise-Heart-Disease-Project) in 1977 [25] showed a significant gap in the cumulative mortality rate over three years for patients after MI who participated in regular exercise as compared to the

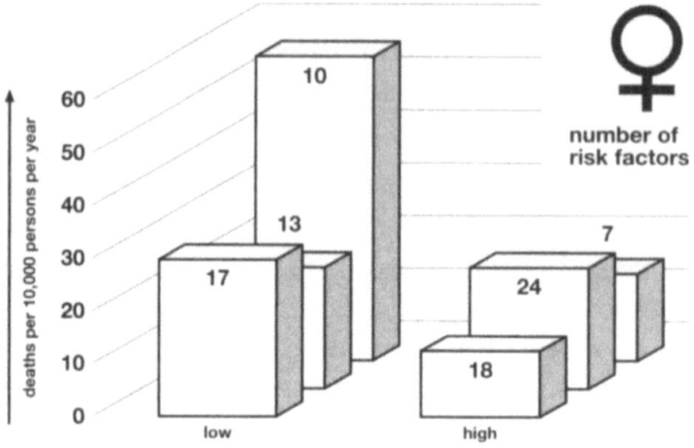

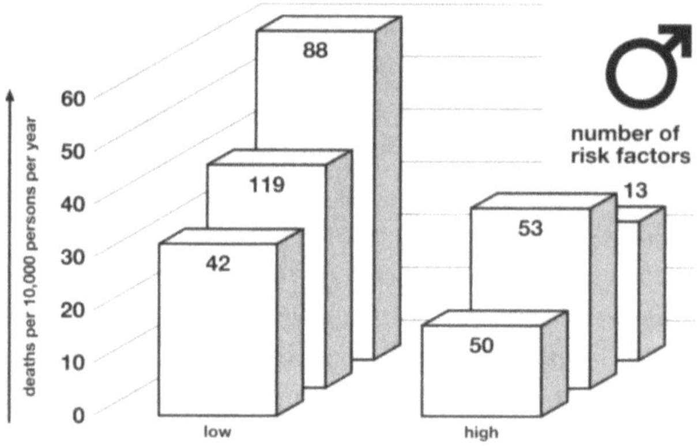

Figs. 2 a+b Cardiorespiratory fitness.
Relationship between physical fitness and mortality for 7,080 women (Fig. 2a) and 15,341 men (Fig. 2b). The left columns represent patients with a low fitness level and the right columns represent patients with a high fitness level. The different columns within each group mark the number of risk factors. It is apparent that men as well as women with low physical fitness levels and multiple risk factors have a significantly higher mortality risk than patients with high fitness level [2].

sedentary group. Regular physical exercise also increased endurance. In addition, it could also be shown that – after 12 months of regular intensive endurance training – the ST-segment depression in the stress ECG at a submaximal stress level was significantly lower (Fig. 3) [7]. Further clinical studies proved that regular physical exercise reduces risk factors and can, in combination with life-style changes, slow down progression of the coronary stenoses, or even lead to regression, and improve physical performance. In the "Lifestyle-Heart-Study", patients were randomized into two groups and followed-up for a maximum of two years, and underwent invasive diagnostic procedures at the beginning and end of the study to determine the coronary status. The control group was treated in the standard manner. The intervention group was asked to change their lifestyle, with a focus on low-fat vegetarian diet, abstainence from smoking, engaging in endurance training and stress reduction techniques. This group improved their endurance limit to 37 minutes/day in comparison to the control group, with 20 minutes/day. The number of angina attacks decreased from 4.4 to 0.4 attacks per week for the

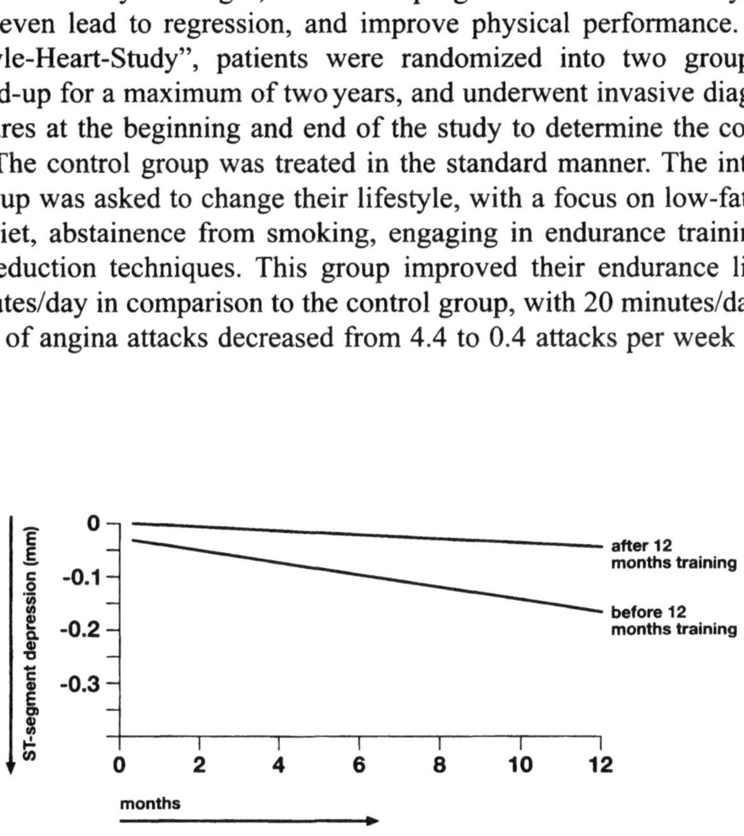

Fig. 3 Decrease in ST-segment depression: after 12 months of intensive exercise training.
Significant decrease in ischemic ST-segment depression during submaximal bicycle exercise training before and after 12 months of intensive training in patients with coronary artery disease: from 0.20 ± 0.04 mV to 0.16 ± 0.08 mV ($p < 0.01$) [7].

intervention group, whereas the control group reported an increase from 2.4 to 6.2 attacks per week. The intervention group experienced a reduction in cholesterol of 229 mg/dl to 178 mg/dl, while the control group's cholesterol decreased only from 248 mg/dl to 229 mg/dl. The angiographic findings were very significant: in the intervention group, 86 % of 195 stenoses showed no signs of progression, or were reported as regressing, whereas 53 % of the control group showed a progression [28]. The randomized Heidelberg intervention study followed 113 patients with CHD over a period of six years. The study also demonstrated an increase in exercise capacity, from 166 to 212 watts. 19 % of the patients in the intervention group exhibited a regression of stenosis. Further analysis revealed that most patients in the group experiencing regression used more energy through physical activity, on average 1,800 to 2,000 calories/week. The physical endurance of patients using between 1,400 and 1,500 calories per week on physical activity improved, but there was no change in coronary status. A progression in coronary sclerosis was seen significantly more frequently in the group that used only 1,000 calories per week (Fig. 4) [26].

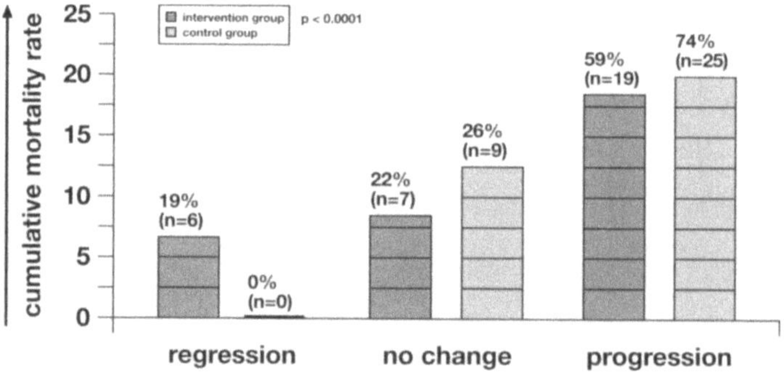

Fig. 4 Nitrates and physical exercise: change in relative diameter of stenosis. Regression or attenuated progression of relative diameter of stenosis in coronary angiography after 6 years [26].

A meta-analysis of 22 studies by O'Connor showed that the total mortality rate for physically fit MI patients could be reduced by approximately 20 %, a result comparable to the effects of β-adrenergic blocker therapy [27]. In February a review entitled "Primary and secondary prevention of coronary heart disease: What can we afford?" appeared in the German medical journal "Zeitschrift für Kardiologie". The authors compared the costs and effects of β-adrenergic blockers, ASS, and HMG-CoA reductase inhibitors on morbidity based on a meta-analysis of available data. The most inexpensive therapy – regular physical exercise – was not mentioned and is presented here attached to the bottom of Table 1 [17, 11].

Table 1 Primary and secondary prevention of coronary heart disease: What can we afford? [17]

Drug	reduction of coronary events (%)	meta-analysis	cost/patient/ year (DM)
beta-blocking agents	20	Prog. Cardio-vascular Dis. 27 (1985) 335	310.00 (100 mg Meto-prodol/Atenolol
aspirin	25	Br. Med. J. 296 (1998) 320	36.00 (100 mg acetylsa-licylic acid)
HMG-CoA-reductase-inhibitor	24–31	Internist 39 (1998) 987	1,197.00 to 2,390.00 (20–40 mg simvastatin/pravasta-tin)
cardiovascular training	20	Circulation 8 (1989) 234	—

In conclusion, patients in the post-MI period also benefit from a regular exercise program. It leads to:

- reduced mortality
- reduction of risk factors
- reduced progression, or regression, of coronary stenosis

- increased efficiency of cardiac function
- increased endurance
- fewer angina pectoris attacks
- (improved left ventricular function)

Importance of nitrates for exercise training in coronary heart disease

Oral application of short-acting or long-acting nitrates, as well as transdermal application of nitrates, leads to:

- reduction of preload and afterload
- dilation of coronary arteries, especially greater coronary arteries
- inhibition of platelet aggregation
- reduction of angina pectoris attacks
- increased or higher degree of endurance
- decrease of ischemia-induced ST-segment depression in stress or endurance ECG
- lower wall motion score in stress echocardiogram

Several studies showed that the use of nitrates improved the endurance capacity of patients. Nitroglycerin spray used prior to exercise increased the excercise duration by 30 % before the onset of angina symptoms and reduced the ST-segment depression from 2.1 ± 1.0 mm to 1.3 ± 0.5 mm (Fig. 5) [11, 14, 16].

Thadani et al. reported improved endurance for up to 8 hours for varying nitrate dosages. However, higher nitrate doses failed to further increase the effect [34]. Transdermal application of nitroglycerin increased endurance as well (on average by 35 seconds). A larger study, however, showed that a significant difference could no longer be found after 8 weeks. Higher nitroglycerin doses did not result in an improvement in endurance either. The number of angina events was reduced from > 7 to 2 [30]. Nitroglycerin therapy also increased the ejection fraction from 36 % to 48 %, and there was a corresponding reduction in stress-induced wall motion abnormalities after a dose of

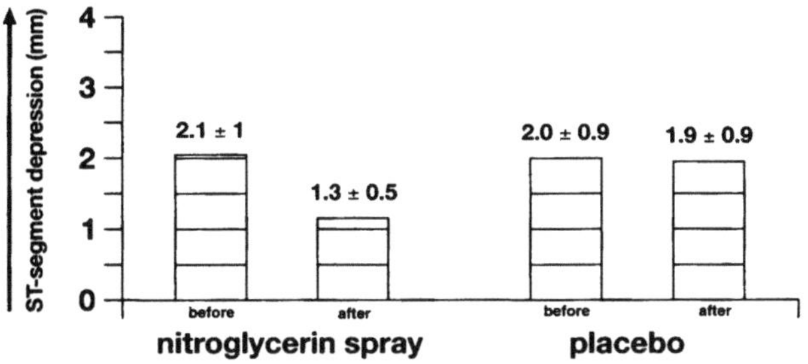

Fig. 5 Decrease of excercise-induced ST-segment depression after application of nitroglycerin spray.
After application of nitroglycerin spray there is a significant decrease of ST-segment depression at the highest exercise level from 2.1 mm to 1.3 mm; as expected, the placebo treatment did not effect any change [14].

0.4 mg nitroglycerin [4]. With appropriate therapy and a controlled exercise program, coronary heart disease patients can exercise symptom-free and with less anxiety.

The prophylactic use of nitrates is covered in another chapter. The prophylactic use of nitrate spray or capsules (sublingual) can improve endurance and stress capacity. Despite the positive results of nitrate therapy, however, nitrate tolerance must be considered. Several studies have shown that endurance increases after acute ISDN/ISMN treatment and with increasing nitrate dosage. Yet, in chronic oral and transdermal nitrate therapy, with constant nitrate levels, endurance and ST-segment depression returned almost to the initial value [1, 22, 32]. Changes in dosage schedules or intermittent application can preserve the effects of nitrate therapy; with the drawback that 24-hour anti-ischemic protection is no longer provided.

Other new therapy approaches, like the concomitant application of antioxidants such as vitamin C, N-acetylcysteine, or vasoconstrictors, could increase the importance of nitrates in the treatment of CHD in the future. Combination therapy with N-acetylcysteine or vitamin C showed a significantly lower

ST-segment depression in the stress ECG; but the endurance time and the length of time until onset of angina pectoris symptoms remained unchanged [36, 5].

Nitrates in chronic CHD and heart failure

Animal tests have indicated that nitrates could prevent left ventricular dilation as well as expansion of the infarction area [21]. However, the use of nitrates after myocardial infarction is still controversial, since there has been no large study showing a positive effect on remodeling. A subgroup analysis in the V-Heft-II-study showed that the combination of hydralazine and nitrates had a positive effect on mortality [38]. In the GISSI-3 study, the positive effect of six weeks of combination therapy (after MI), consisting of a GTN transdermal patch and lisinopril was measurable after six months. Older patients seem to benefit most from this combination [9, 10]. Additional nitrates (in the form of slow release isosorbide mononitrate) were also used in the ISIS-4 study, and again only slight positive effects on mortality were seen in the nitrate-treated group [12].

However, there can be no doubt about the positive effect of nitrate therapy combined with either ACE inhibitors or beta blockers on hemodynamics and symptoms. A recently published review in the European Heart Journal reported that, across Europe, 45 % of patients with chronic heart failure are treated with nitrates [35]. Past studies involving patients with ischemic heart failure showed that ISDN, as well as ISMN significantly reduce left and right ventricular filling pressure and systemic and pulmonary vascular resistance, and also increase cardiac output [15]. Slow release nitrate preparations showed advantages over nitroglycerin. There was also an increase in physical fitness with nitrate therapy. A long-term study by Elkayam showed that, in patients with severe heart failure, (NYHA III-IV) increased nitrate doses, intermittent application and additional application of hydralazine prevented nitrate tolerance and improved cardiac performance [31, 6, 8]. A small study involving patients with CHD and heart failure and pre-existing nitrate tolerance showed an improvement in hemodynamics after oral application of 50 mg captopril

[33]. However, none of these studies showed a significant effect of organic nitrates on morbidity and mortality of patients with MI and heart failure.

Established methods for assessment of the degree of ischemia after physical exercise or drug therapy for coronary artery disease are stress ECG, myocardial scintigraphy, and coronary angiography. Recently, magnetic resonance imaging and electron beam computed tomography have been used for diagnostic and therapy evaluation. Stress echocardiography is a non-invasive technique that is also suitable for assessing anti-ischemic effects of drugs. Eight days after ISDN therapy a significant decrease in wall motion score of 2.5 ± 2.5 compared with placebo, was reported (Fig. 6) [20].

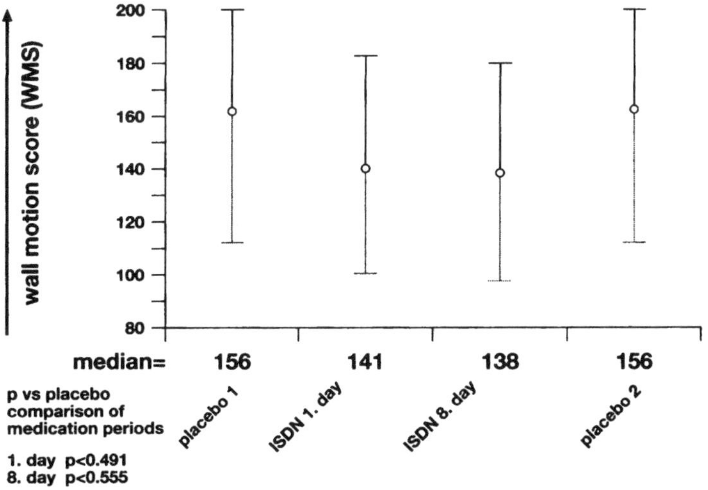

Fig. 6 Exercise echocardiography: wall motion score – placebo/nitrate. Change of wall motion score in exercise echocardiogram during therapy with ISDN or placebo under comparable maximum exertion [20].

The following case history illustrates the clinical use of stress ECG and stress echocardiography in assessing the endurance of a patient with severe chronic CAD after bypass surgery and repeated catheterizations with and without full medication with 2 puffs of nitrolingual spray prior to exercise:

Case history: F. T., date of birth: 01.22.1946

risk factors: hypercholesterolemia, arterial hypertension

angina pectoris: since fall 1991 despite use of ASS, bisoprolol fumarate, nitrate, molsidomine, HMG-CoA-reductase inhibitor

aortocoronary bypass 2/92: internal mammary artery to anterior ventricular artery, vein to right coronary artery, sequential vein to CX and RD

increasing angina pectoris symptoms since 8/92

abnormal exercise ECG 9/92

coronary angiography 11/99: severe stenosis of internal mammary artery anastomosis

PTCA 12/92 of stenoses of anterior ventricular artery and descending artery

persisting angina pectoris

PTCA 1/93 of stenoses of anterior ventricular artery

PTCA 3/93 of peripheral stenoses of anterior ventricular artery and descending artery

rotablation of recurrent RCA stenosis 10/93

PTCA of recurrent RCA stenosis next to bypass anastomosis 11/93

check coronary angiography 7/94: open bypasses, insignificant residual stenoses

no symptoms; exercise ECG normal 9/94!

12/97 again angina symptoms and pathologic exercise ECG

coronary angiography 10/98: severe stenosis of distal internal mammary artery anastomosis, proximal occlusion of anterior and posterior interventricular artery, bypasses clear, good left ventricular function

myocardial scintigraphy 10/98: normal

conservative treatment

stress ECG without medication abnormal at 75 watts

stress ECG after nitroglycerin normal up to 125 watts

stress echocardiography normal after nitroglycerin

(Figs. 7 and 8)

Summary

Regular, intensive exercise has a significant positive effect in the primary prevention of coronary heart disease. Physical exercise, in the form of individualized endurance training for CAD patients results in: reduced mortality, reduction of risk factors, decreased progression and/or regression of coronary sclerosis, improved efficiency of cardiac function, improved left ventricular function, improved physical endurance and improved, angina-free work capacity.

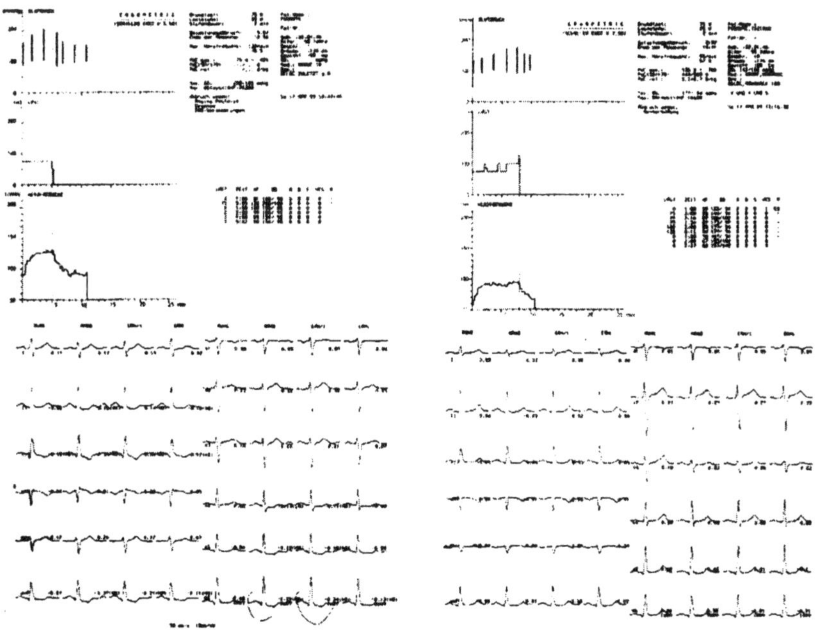

Fig. 7 Case history F. T.: Exercise ECG without and with medication.
Clearly visible ST-segment depression in II, III, V5 and V6 at 75 watts in the exercise ECG without medication (left). The patients also complained about angina symptoms. After 2 puffs of nitroglycerin spray, in addition to maximum antianginose medication, the patient can exercise up to 125 without ST-segment depression and angina symptoms (right). The test was stopped due to physical exhaustion.

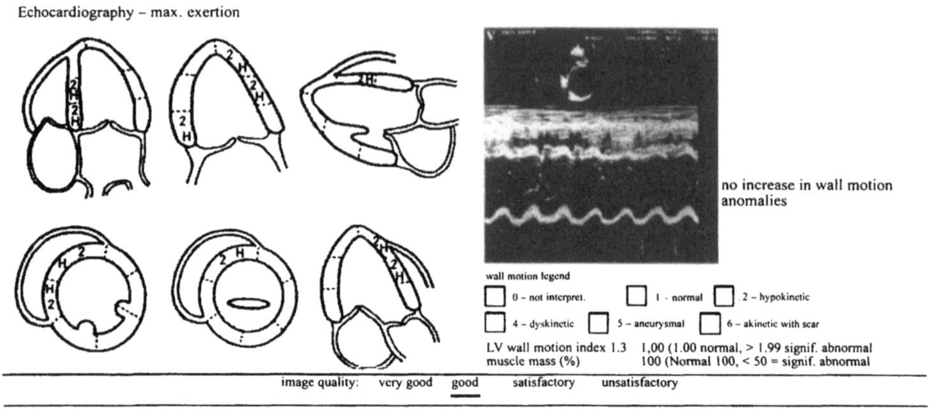

Fig. 8 Exercise echocardiography.
There are no additional wall motion anomalies in the exercise echocardiography at 125 watts with optimum medication.

Additional use of nitrates (long-acting and short-acting nitrates: buccal/sublingual/oral/transdermal) decreases the number of angina attacks in coronary heart disease patients and increases the duration and degree of physical endurance and improves the quality of life. These effects can be recorded non-invasively as a decrease in ischemic ST-segment depression in endurance ECG or as a decrease in wall motion anomalies in stress echocardiogram. Thus, the endurance limit of patients with CHD can be assessed repeatedly and individually adjusted.

References

[1] Abshagen, U.: Kontrollierte klinische Studien zur Toleranzentwicklung und Dosierungsprobleme der Nitrattherapie. Herz 21 (Suppl. I) (1996) 23–30.

[2] Blair, S., K. Cooper, L. Gettman et al.: Changes in coronary heart disease risk factors associated with increased treadmill time in 753 men. Am. J. Epidemiol. (1983) 352–359.

[3] Blair, S., J. Kampert, H. Kohl et al.: Influences of cardiorespiratory fitness and other precursors on cardiovascular disease and all-cause mortality in men and women. JAMA 276 (1996) 205–210.
[4] Borer, J., S. Bacharach, M. Green et al.: Effect of nitroglycerin on exercise-induced abnormalities of left ventricular regional function and ejection fraction in coronary artery disease. Circulation 57 (1978) 314–320.
[5] Boesgaard, S., J. Aldershvile, F. Petersen et al.: Continous oral N-acetylcysteine treatment and development of nitrate tolerance in patients with stable angina pectoris. J. Cardiovasc. Pharmacol. (1991) 889–893.
[6] Elkayam, U., A. Roth, A. Mehra: Randomized study to evaluate the relation between oral isosorbide dinitrate dosing interval and the development of early tolerance to its effect on left ventricular filling pressure in patients with chronic heart failure. Circulation 84 (1991) 2040–2048.
[7] Eshani, A., G. Heath, J. Hagberg et al.: Effects of 12 month of intensive exercise training on ischemic ST-segment depression in patients with coronary artery disease. Circulation 64 (1981) 1116–1124.
[8] Franciosa, J., A. Goldsmith, J. Cohn: Contrasting immediate and long-term effects of isosorbid dinitrate on exercise capacity in congestive heart failure. Am. J. Cardiol. 69 (1980) 559–566.
[9] GISSI-3: Effects of lisinopril and transdermalglyceryl trinitrate single or together on 6-week mortality and ventricular function after acute myocardial function. Gruppo Italiano per lo Studio Sopravivenzy nell'Infarto Miocardio. Lancet 343 (1994) 1115–1122.
[10] GISSI-3 Investigators: Six month effects of early treatment with lisinopril and nitroglycerin withdrawn 6-weeks after myocardial infarction. The GISSI-3 results in elderly patients. Circulation 90 (1994) 1–325 (abstr.).
[11] Gohlke, H.: Nutzen und Risiken der körperlichen Aktivität bei Patienten mit koronarer Herzerkrankung. Wien. Klin. Wochenschr. 107 (1995) 760–765.
[12] ISIS Collaborative Group: ISIS-4: Randomized study of oral isosorbide mononitrate in over 50,000 patients with suspected acute myocardial infarction. Circulation 88 (1993) I–394.
[13] Judgutt, B.: Effects of nitrate therapy on left ventricular remodeling and function. Am. J. Cardiol. 72 (1993) 161G–181G.
[14] Kimchi, A., G. Lee, E. Amsterdam et al.: Increased exercise tolerance after nitroglycerin oral spray: a new and effective therapeutic modality in angina pectoris. Circulation 67 (1983) 124–127.
[15] Kodja, G.: Hämodynamische Wirkungen organischer Nitrate. MMP 21 (1998) 9–15.
[16] Kolenda, K.-D.: Stellenwert von Glyceroltrinitrat im Rahmen der Bewegungstherapie. Fortschr. Med. 116 (1998) 65–70.

[17] Kübler,W., J. Kreuzer: Primäre und sekundäre Prävention der koronaren Herzerkrankung: Was können wir uns leisten? Z. Kardiol. 88 (1999) 85–89.

[18] Kupper, W., E. Krasemann, A. Rotermund et al.: Ergebnisse von Kursen zur Primärprävention von Herz-Kreislauferkrankungen. Herz/Kreisl. 27 (1995) 198–202.

[19] Leary, T.: Coronary spasm as a possible factor in producing sudden death. Am. Heart J. 10 (1935) 338–342.

[20] Leischik, R., O. Adamczewski, S. Pötter et al.: Belastungsechokardiographie – ein neuer Test zur Erfassung einer antiischämischen Medikamentenwirkung. Z. Kardiol. 84 (1999) 621–632.

[21] McDonald, K., G. Francis, J. Matthew et al.: Long-term oral nitrate therapy prevents chronic ventricular remodeling in the dog. JACC 21 (1993) 514–522.

[22] Mehmel, H.: Nitrate in der Therapie der koronaren Herzerkrankung. Neue Aspekte nach 100 Jahren klinischer Praxis. Therapiewoche 44 Sonderheft September (1994) 13–16.

[23] Mittleman, M., M. Maclure, G. Tofler et al.: Triggering of acute myocardial infarction by heavy physical exertion. Protection against triggering by regular exertion. N. Engl. J. Med. 329 (1993) 1677–1683.

[24] Morris, J., D. Clayton, M. Everitt et al.: Exercise in leisure-time: coronary attack and death rates. Br. Heart J. 68 (1990) 325–334.

[25] Naughton, J.: Exercise and myocardial infarction. The National Exercise and Heart Disease Project; an overview. US DHSS PHS, NIH 1977.

[26] Niebauer, J., R. Hambrett, T. Velich et al.: Attenuated progression of coronary artery disease after 6 years of multifactorial risk intervention. Role of physical exercise. Circulation 8 (1997) 2534–254.

[27] O'Connor, G., I. Buring, S. Yusuf et al.: An overview of randomized trials of rehabilitation with exercise after myocardial infarction. Circulation 8 (1989) 234–244.

[28] Ornish, D., L. Scherwitz, W. Armstrong et al.: Können Veränderungen des Lebenstils die koronare Herzkrankheit rückgängig machen? Die "Lifestyle-Heart"-Studie. Lancet, Deutsche Ausgabe 4 (1990) 591–596.

[29] Paffenbarger, R., R. Hyde, R. Wing et al.: The association of changes in physical activity level and other lifestyle characteristics with mortality in men. N. Engl. J. Med. 328 (1993) 538–545.

[30] Poorvin, D. on behalf of the Steering Committee, Transdermal Nitroglycerin Cooperative Study: Acute and chronic antianginal efficacy of continous twenty-four-hour application of transdermal nitroglycerin. Am. J. Cardiol. 68 (1991) 1263–1273.

[31] Rabinovitz, B.: Hemodynamic effect of oral isosorbide-5-mononitrate and dinitrate in patients with ischemic heart failure. Clin. Cardiol. 10 (1987) 603–608.

[32] Silber, S.: Nitrates: why and how should they be used today? Current status of the clinical usefulness of nitroglycerin, isosorbide dinitrate and isosorbide-5-mononitrate. Europ. J. Clin. Pharmacol. 38 Suppl 1 (1990) 35–51.

[33] Störk, T., H. Eichstätt, M. Möckel et al: Hemodynamic action of captopril in coronary patients with heart failure tolerant to nitroglycerin. Clin. Cardiol. 20 (1997) 999–1004.

[34] Thadani, U., H. Fung, A. Darke et al.: Oral isosorbide dinitrate in the treatment of angina pectoris. Dose-response relationship and duration of action during acute therapy. Circulation 62 (1980) 491–502.

[35] Veldhuisen, D., A. Charlesworth, H. Crijns et al.: Differences in drug treatment of chronic heart failure between European countries. Eur. Heart J. 20 (1999) 666–672.

[36] Watanabe, H., M. Kakihana, S. OhTsuka et al.: Randomized, double-blind, placebo-controlled study of the preventive effect of supplemental oral vitamin C on attenuation of the development of nitrate tolerance. JACC 31 (1998) 1323–1329.

[37] Willich, S., R. Arnzt, H. Löwel et al.: Trimm-Studiengruppe (Berlin-Augsburg) Belastungssituation beim akuten Myokardinfarkt: Die Rolle von körperlicher Anstrengung und ungewöhnlichen Lebensereignissen. Z. Kardiol. 83 (1994) 423–430.

[38] Ziesche, S., F. Cobb, J. Cohn et al.: Hydralazine and isosorbide dinitrate combination improves exercise tolerance in heart failure. Results from V-HeFT I and V-HeFT II. The V-HeFT VA Cooperative Studies Group. Circulation 87 (1993) VI 56–64.

Rehabilitation in Germany compared with other European countries

P. Mathes

The annual number of new patients with cardiovascular disease in Germany is in the range of 700,000 to 900,000. According to the latest data from the MONICA study this figure includes some 281,000 myocardial infarctions. The total mortality within the first 28 days, including prehospital mortality, is about 50 %. Some 20 % of all hospitalized patients will undergo a PTCA within 28 days and approximately 5 % have a bypass operation [4, 8].

These data show that coronary heart disease is one of the leading medical problems in Germany. It is responsible for 8.3 million hospital days and 184,000 fatalities per year. Over the last few years, the number of heart catheterizations, dilatations, stent implantations, and bypass operations has risen, making it an economical problem, too. In 1993 the cost for inpatient treatment was 3.6 billion Deutschmarks and the costs for prescriptions and outpatient treatment added up to 3.1 billion Deutschmarks. Thus, 2.8 % of all direct expenses for therapy were spent on coronary heart disease [4]. Apart from that there are considerable indirect costs caused by disability, impairment, and premature death. Keeping in mind that diagnostic procedures and therapy have increased as well as the possibilities of secondary prevention by means of drug treatment, one can assume that these costs should have increased considerably in the meantime.

Rehabilitation, as defined by the WHO as well as by the VDR, has always had one primary goal: reduction of unnecessary invalidism and re-integration of patients into their workplace and social environment. Yet, from the first day on, this goal has been a point of controversy in Germany [7]. Its protagonists claim that rehabilitation is a humanitarian effort that pays tribute not only to somatic but also to psychosocial models of disease and coping with it, thus giving medicine a new direction. Antagonists, however, denounced it as a waste of resources marked by high hopes but little results and by an absence of solid data, infringing the principles of evidence-based medicine [3].

Compared with this situation, rehabilitation is looked upon far less emotionally in other West European countries, maybe because it is primarily based on outpatient treatment, and therefore uses up a smaller part of the available resources.

How did this development come about?

The modern principles of rehabilitation of cardiovascular disorders rest on two pillars:

1. The psychosomatic (or somatopsychic) approach, which sees the risk factor model as a sequel of an intrapersonal autoaggression.

   Keywords: infarction personality
   managers' disease
   type A personality
   autoaggressive behavior

   Hans Selye, Julius Raab, Meyer-Friedman and Ray Rosenman are amongst the well-known advocates in the USA, as are Max Halhuber and Kurt König in Germany.

2. The principle of appropriate exercise therapy, which goes back to the work done by Paul Dudley White. Originally, any kind of heart disorder was automatically treated with rest and reduced physical activity. However, White was able to prove for the first time that appropriate exercise therapy is useful in treatment as well as in prevention of heart disorders. Kenneth Cooper in the USA and Peter Beckmann, Reindell, Hollmann, and Rost in Germany further extended on this method.

   Early mobilization, early discharge from hospital, and reduced hospital time in myocardial infarction are developments based on this model and the importance of these should not be underestimated. Large studies such as GISSI, TIMI, among others, show that patients with myocardial infarction should be discharged 5 to 7 days after the incident. However, recent studies of the Arbeitsgemeinschaft leitender kardiologischer Krankenhausärzte (ALKK) in Germany show that patients with myocardial infarction are still hospitalized for 21 days with a mortality of 15 % during this interval and 12.5 % during the following year. These figures are much higher than one would expect on the basis of the GISSI and TIMI studies (MITRA and MIR involving some 22,000 patients).

The data from MONICA [4, 8] show that, in 1993, 65 % of all patients with MI received rehabilitation therapy, so-called follow-up treatment. For gainfully employed patients, this figure was even higher (90 %). Some 20 % continued their rehabilitation in a coronary group. The Arbeiterrentenversicherung (a pension fund for manual workers) paid for 69,823 rehabilitation treatments for cardiovascular disorders, whereas the Bundesanstalt für Angestellte (the federal pension fund) paid for 49,882 treatments. Based on average costs of 6,000.00 Deutschmarks per treatment, the total costs can be estimated at more than 700 million Deutschmarks.

Over the last few years cost-saving measures due to an unfavorable economic development have reduced the number of rehabilitation treatments; in 1997 the total number of follow-up treatments was 53,256 (20,562 for the Arbeiterrentenversicherung and 32,694 for the Bundesanstalt für Angestellte) while the number of patients who survived a myocardial infarction remained constant at 140,000. On the basis of these 1993 figures we have to assume that the vast majority of patients with MI receive no follow-up rehabilitation treatment.

The integration of the psychosomatic model and the exercise-based therapy in Germany created a very intensive early rehabilitation which is rather expensive. In other Western European countries, outpatient treatment based primarily on exercise therapy, developed e.g., the Club de Coeur Santé in France and the Coronary Groups in Great Britain. There are a number of well-documented studies showing that this approach is as efficient as the intensive early rehabilitation in hospitals in Germany. However, patients in these countries complain about a lack of follow-up rehabilitation. They find it hard to understand why they are rushed to the hospital where they are treated as an emergency in the coronary care unit just to be told one week later that they can go home and lead a risk-free life again. These patients suffer from a deep-seated sense of insecurity; the time up to when they are accepted into a rehabilitation unit (for security reasons, they cannot accept a patient until 4 weeks after an infarction) is a very traumatic period for them [1].

A study recently published in France (PREVENIR) involved 1,456 patients that where admitted with an acute myocardial infarction to one of 77 cardiologic centers. 24% of these patients took part in an outpatient rehabilitation program. In Ireland the percentage of patients taking part in rehabilitation programs is below 10%; there is no information available from Great Britain. However, it is realistic to assume an even lower percentage.

The numbers for Italy are completely different. In 1996 there were 114 cardiologic rehabilitation centers, 65 in the North, 26 in the center, and 23 in the South. Among them are 10 centers for in-hospital treatment only, 66 centers run outpatient programs, and 38 centers offer in-hospital and outpatient treatment. The total number of patients entering a formal rehabilitation program was 37,049 for 1996. Most of them lived in the North (26,360), with 7,007 in the center and 4,500 in the South. The majority of patients (25,540, i.e., 66%) took part in in-hospital rehabilitation [2].

In light of the fact that Mediterranean countries have a lower infarction incidence, it can be assumed that a higher percentage of patients receives in-hospital rehabilitation compared with Germany.

In Germany, sufficient provision with rehabilitation units allows for a comprehensive care of patients with MI and coronary heart disorders. However, this does not come cheap. The change of environment and the attractive scenery surrounding most rehabilitation centers are frequent reasons for patients to enter a rehabilitation program. Unfortunately, the basic idea of rehabilitation as "change of lifestyle as a means of secondary prevention" is often overlooked. Most patients embrace this idea only reluctantly, as the changes involve deep alterations in their customary behavior. Thus, the attractive setting of rehabilitation centers is not a luxury but a necessity, as it makes it easier for patients to take part in the programs. It comes as no surprise that ambulatory centers which, as a means of cutting down on health care costs, have been opened in densely populated areas find it hard to compete for patients.

This new model of part in-hospital and part outpatient treatment is based upon the „Kölner Modell“ by Rost [4]. There is no doubt that this model has a lot of advantages: there can be no confusion of vacation with rehabilitation, and the change in lifestyle is at the center of the program, not just a necessary evil spoiling a recreation period. New behavior patterns can be incorporated into everyday life immediately. Relatives, and the whole social environment, including the family physician, can be involved in the rehabilitation process more easily.

Regardless of all these efforts – and of the great differences – the success achieved so far leaves room for more improvement. The EuroAspire study has shown that, for a large proportion of the post-MI population in all European countries, the risk factors were in the suboptimal area, proving that more efforts are necessary in order to make complete use of the potential for secondary prevention.

References

[1] Bethell, H., S. Turner: Management and rehabilitation of the post-infarct-patient. Science Press, London 1996.

[2] Giannuzzi Pantaleo: Survey of Italian Rehabilitation Centers. (Personal communication.)

[3] Held, K.: Die Neuorientierung der kardiologischen Rehabilitation. Münch. Med. Wschr. 141 (1999) 181–184.

[4] Löwel, H., A. Dobson, U. Keil et al.: Coronary heart disease case fatality in 4 countries. Circulation 88 (1993) 2524–2531.

[5] Rost, R.: Der Bedarf an ambulanten kardiologischen Anschlußrehabilitationen in einem großstädtischen Ballungsgebiet. Z. Kardio. 88 (1999) 34–43.

[6] Troche, C.J., B. Tacke, B. Hinzpeter et al.: Costeffectivnes of primary and secondary prevention in cardiovascular diseases. Eur. Heart J. 19 (1998) Suppl. C, C59–65.

[7] WHO Expert Commitee: Rehabilitation after cardiovascular diseases, WHO Technical Report Series 831 (1993).

[8] Willich, S., H. Löwel et al.: Regionale Unterschiede der Herz-Kreislauf-Mortalität in Deutschland. DÄ 96 (1999) 479–483.

The prophylactic use of glyceryl trinitrate

S. P. Glasser

Introduction

Although the concept of nitroglycerin prophylaxis may be relatively new, nitroglycerin and long acting nitrates have been available for more than a century. The issue of tolerance to these drugs was first raised 100 years ago, and remains a topic of considerable interest and controversy. Tolerance remains one of the most important limiting factors in the clinical use of long acting nitrates. However, tolerance is not an issue with the short acting preparations. Short acting nitroglycerin preparations are utilized to relieve the pain of an already established attack of angina, or to prevent an attack of angina prior to an activity known to precipitate it. It is this latter use which is the subject of the following review.

It is unclear when the first suggestion for the prophylactic use of nitroglycerin was made, but Aranow in 1973 stated: "In my experience, nitroglycerin is most useful as an antianginal drug when administered 2–3 minutes before performance of activities (...) in which an anginal attack may be precipitated" [1]. However, at about the same time, Stipe and Fink said that "traditionally, amyl nitrate and nitroglycerin have been used to terminate the acute attack; however, the efficacy of organic nitrates in preventing attacks remains undecided" [15]. Stipe and Fink also reviewed the literature from 1952–1972 and identified 91 articles relating to the efficacy of immediate use nitroglycerin prophylaxis. They found that 30 of the 91 studies failed to demonstrate effectiveness, and that this observation was particularly true with the more rigorous scientific studies. However, the details of the studies reviewed were not presented [15]. In 1994, Thadani and Lipicky stated that "sublingual NTG tablets or spray (...) increase angina free walking time (...) when administered just prior to engaging in short-term physical or emotional stress, as prophylaxis against anticipated angina" [16].

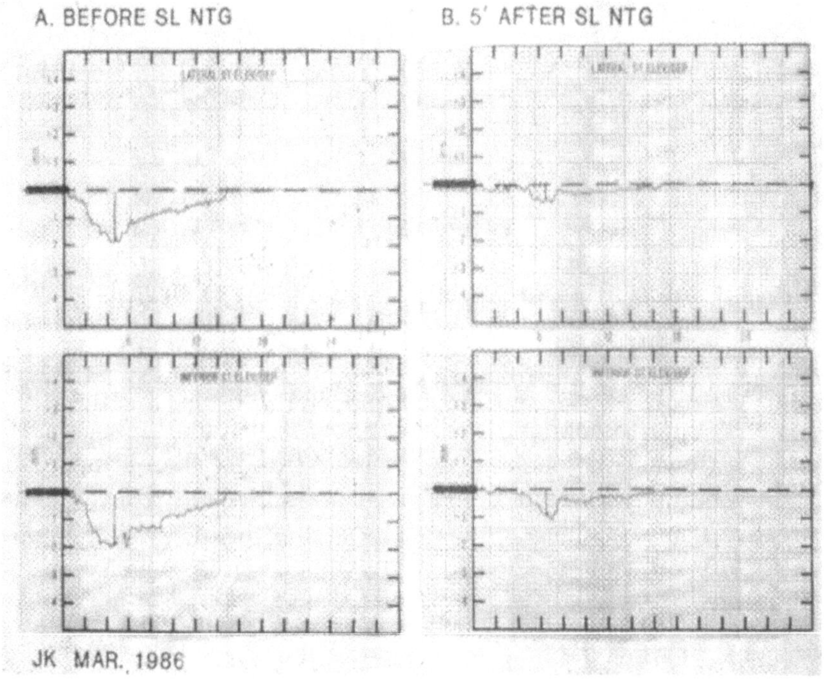

Fig. 1 An histogram of the exercise-induced lateral and inferior ST-segment deviation from a patient with chronic stable angina pectoris, before and 5 minutes after receiving sublingual NTG. The upright sharp line designates the end of exercise. Note the longer exercise time after NTG and the marked reduction in ST-segment depression.

The acute effects of nitroglycerin are impressive in a number of clinical settings. Fig. 1 represents a histogram of the ST-segment response during and after exercise in a 55 year old male with chronic stable angina, who underwent exercise tolerance testing (as part of a clinical trial) before and 5 minutes after receiving 0.4 mg of NTG sublingually.

Despite longer exercise time after NTG use, the ischemic response to exercise was abolished; and, exercise was terminated due to fatigue rather that angina. Gage et al. may explain how this improved response was accomplished [7]. In their study of coronary artery diameter in response to exercise, the normal vessel segment dilated in response to submaximal and maximal exercise, while the abnormal (diseased) segment constricted (a paradoxical response) [7]. Nitroglycerin, administered acutely, further dilated the normal coronary artery segment and reversed the paradoxic vasoconstriction in the diseased segment [7].

Acute hemodynamic effects of sublingual (SL) nitroglycerin

Thadani and Parker evaluated the influence of SL NTG during supine and upright exercise in patients with angina pectoris [17]; and, Chevigne et al. studied the hemodynamic response of glyceryl trinitrate (GTN or NTG) in a spray at rest and during supine and sitting exercise [2, 3]. Thadani and Parker found that NTG induced a fall in systolic blood pressure and a rise in heart rate which was more pronounced in the standing than in a sitting position [17]. Chevigne et al. found that in the supine position, in subjects with compensated hearts, GTN induced a fall in right atrial and capillary wedge pressure, but had no effect on heart rate or cardiac output [2]. In a sitting exercise study, 15 patients with class II or III angina, all of whom had a normal resting pulmonary wedge pressure, were studied [3]. Four minutes after the administration of NTG, heart rate increased by 13 %, while cardiac and systolic indices decreased by about 13 %. Right atrial pressure, capillary wedge pressure, systemic systolic and mean pressures decreased by 36.5, 48, 19 and 15 % respectively. During exercise, GTN decreased right and left ventricular filling pressures and systemic vascular resistence compared with placebo (Fig. 2).

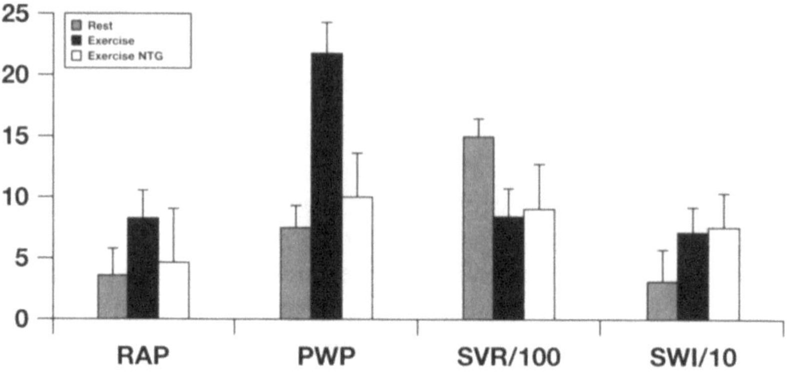

Fig. 2 An adaptation of the hemodynamic response to sublingual NTG spray at rest, after exercise without NTG pre-treatment, and after exercise with NTG pre-treatment. Note the favorable diminution in exercise-induced right arterial pressure (RAP), pulmonary capillary wedge pressure (PWP), systemic vascular resistance (SVR), and stroke work index (SWI) following pre-treatment with NTG.

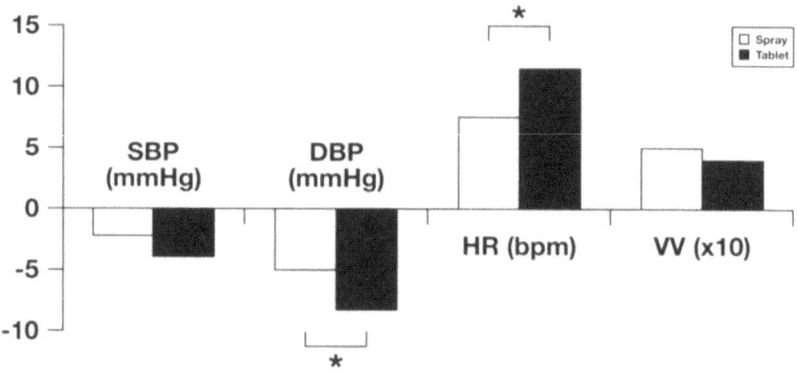

Fig. 3 Comparison of the venodilatory effects of sublingual NTG spray vs. sublingual NTG tablets in healthy subjects. There is a greater reduction in systolic and diastolic blood pressure (SBP, DBP), but with reduced venous volume in treated subjects.

The combined effects on preload and afterload would likely improve subendocardial muscle oxygenation.

In comparing the hemodynamic and venodilatory (determined by plethysmography) effects of NTG spray versus tablets, Fanelli studied 14 healthy volunteers [5]. There were slight differences in heart rate and diastolic blood pressure but no differences in venous volume (Fig. 3).

In addition, the time course of effect was nearly identical between the spray and tablets [5].

Antianginal and antiischemic effects

Kimchi et al. evaluated the prophylactic antianginal efficacy of nitroglycerin oral spray in 20 patients with angiographically documented coronary artery disease and stable angina pectoris (Fig. 4) [10].

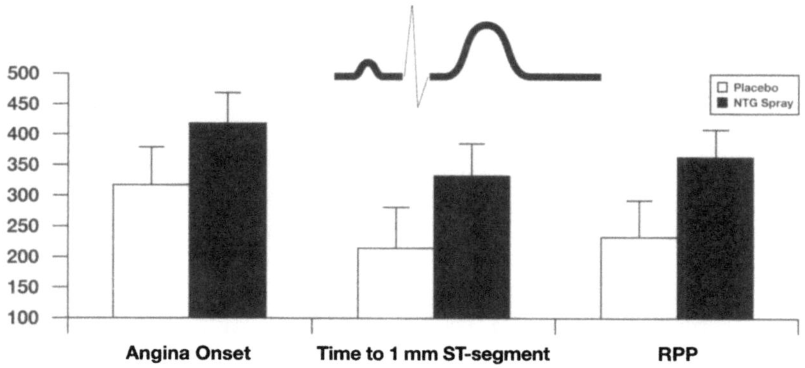

Fig. 4 The effect of pre-treatment sublingual NTG spray compared to placebo on exercise induced EKG and hemodynamic variables. Note prolongation in time to angina onset and 1 mm ST-segment deviation and the higher rate-pressure product (RPP) in patients pre-treated with NTG.

The study design was that of a randomized crossover trial involving treadmill exercise testing, comparing placebo to 0.8 mg of NTG sublingual spray. NTG spray delayed the onset of anginal pain during exercise by a mean of 100 + 64 seconds in 13 patients and entirely prevented pain in 7 patients. Furthermore, total exercise duration was increased by 31%, the onset of exercise induced 1 mm ST-segment depression was abolished in six patients and delayed in 14 patients [10].

Parker et al. studied 20 patients with chronic stable exercise induced angina pectoris, in terms of both its hemodynamic and antianginal effects [12]. A relationship with three doses of spray (0.2, 0.4 and 0.8 mg spray) was compared to 0.4 mg of SL NTG. There was a dose-response in the hemodynamic and antianginal effects, and the 0.4 and 0.8 mg spray was similar compared to 0.4 mg SL NTG (Fig. 5) [12].

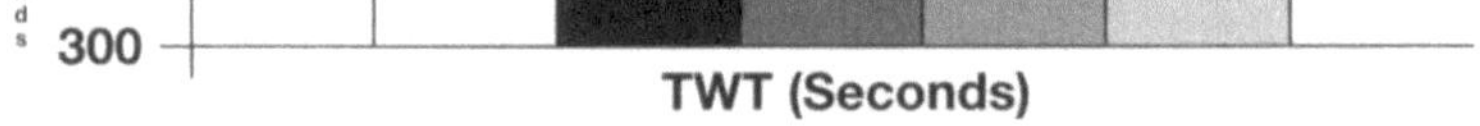

Fig. 5 An evaluation of dose response improvements in treadmill walking time (TWT) of sublingual NTG spray compared to sublingual NTG tablet (0.4 mg).

Detry and Bruce also evaluted both the hemodynamic and antianginal/anti-ischemic effects and demonstrated similar beneficial effects [4] to Parker et al. [12]. Specifically, Detry, and Bruce concluded that nitroglycerin increased MVO2, and lessened angina and evidence of electrocardiographic myocardial ischemia; and that those effects occurred despite the same or higher pressure-rate index.

A question that has been raised regarding the acute effects of SL NTG either as prophylaxis or for aborting the anginal attack, is whether SL NTG is effective in patients already receiving long-acting nitrates. Naito et al. evaluated the effects of SL ISDN in patients receiving sustained ISDN therapy (20 mg q.i.d.) compared to the SL response in those not receiving sustained therapy [11]. They noted that SL ISDN produced less reduction in aortic systolic pressure, and LVEDP, and less dilation of the coronary artery diameter in patients receiving sustained therapy (Fig. 6).

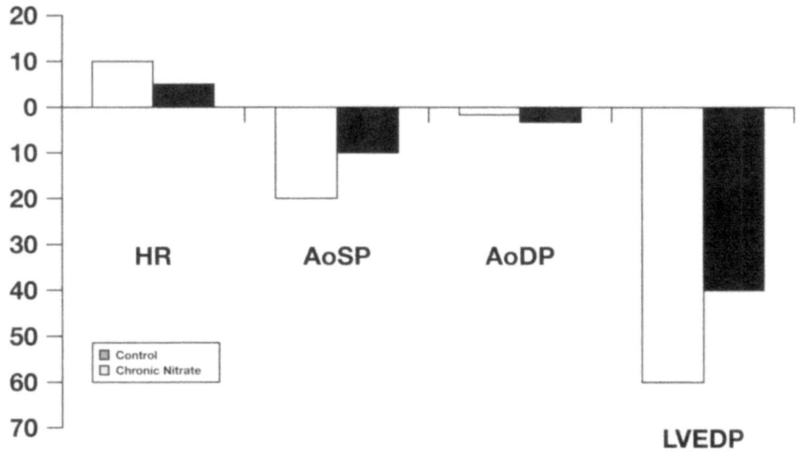

Fig. 6 The effect of sublingual isosorbide dinitrate (ISDN) on hemodynamic parameters in patients not receiving chronic nitrate therapy compared to those having background chronic nitrate therapy. Note that chronic nitrate therapy did diminish (but did not prevent) the beneficial hemodynamic response to sublingual NTG.

In the FDA co-operative study, patients rendered tolerant by virtue of continuous high dose NTG patch therapy, were evaluated relative to their exercise tolerance test in response to SL NTG [14]. Although there was a dose-response decrement in responsiveness to SL NTG, particularly at the lower patch doses, SL NTG responsiveness was still demonstrated.

Another method of determining the vascular effects of NTG is using arterial elasticity measures. Now that non-invasive methods to measure arterial elasticity are available, this is a particularly attractive technique of evaluating vascular integrity in a variety of disease states as well as vascular responsiveness (structural and functional) to a variety of drugs [8, 9]. For example, Feske et al. studied the effects of nipride [6] (NP) and Smulyan the effects of NTG on large and small vessel arterial stiffness [13]. Feske et al. found that NP decreased BP and impedance with a resultant decrease in SVR [6]. However, NP's effect on vascular compliance was more significant than its effect on SVR [6]. Specifically, they noted a 19 % decrease in mean BP, a variable 6 % decrease in SVR; but also a 19 % decrease in proximal and 326 % decrease in distal arterial compliance. Smulyan et al. noted that at any given BP, NTG increased forearm vessel distensibility [13]. We have been evaluating the acute effects of SL NTG on blood vessel stiffness as well as the time course of any changes. A representative example is shown in Fig. 7.

In conclusion, the use of NTG to prevent attacks of angina prior to engaging in an activity that is known to precipitate it, has been recommended for years. Sublingual nitroglycerin preparations have a rapid onset of action, and are suitable for this purpose. The use of SL NTG for the above purpose can be effective even in patients receiving long acting nitrate preparations.

Summary

The beneficial effects of nitrates in patients with ischemic heart disease and congestive heart failure are attributable primarily to relaxation of vascular smooth muscle. Nitrate-induced venodilation reduces venous return and left ventricular preload, thereby decreasing myocardial oxygen demand and

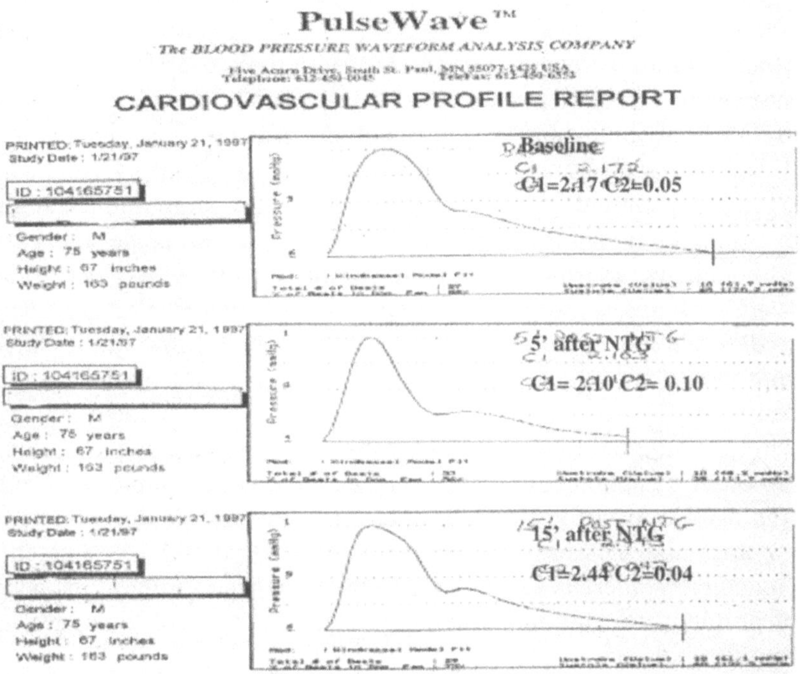

Fig. 7 The pulse wave contour and compliance measurements (C1 and C2 – see text) in response to sublingual NTG. Smaller vessel compliance is beneficially increased within 5 minutes of sublingual NTG. (We are currently evaluating the population-based response and the time course of these changes.)

enhancing left ventricular emptying. Peripheral arterial dilatation produced by nitrates contributes to these beneficial effects by reducing left ventricular afterload. The direct vasodilatory effect of nitrates on the coronary circulation increases myocardial perfusion, thereby improving myocardial oxygen supply. The vasodilatation produced by nitrates depends on the interaction of these compounds with reduced sulfhydryl, or thiol, groups at or near the vascular smooth muscle cell membrane.

Most commonly, long acting nitrates (with the provision of a nitrate free/poor interval to circumvent tolerance) are used; and sublingual nitroglycerin is used to abort acute attacks. The beneficial effect of sublingual nitroglycerin in the prophylactic treatment of angina pectoris is often overlooked. However, since many patients can predict activities which might induce angina, the use of prophylactic sublingual nitroglycerin to prevent acute attacks, has merit. Although the use of prophylactic sublingual nitroglycerin to prevent acute attacks of angina is a not infrequently mentioned strategy, there are few studies that have carefully evaluated this method. Most studies have relied on appropriate surrogate measures of sublingual therapy, such as the effect on hemodynamics and exercise test parameters. There are also few studies comparing sublingual nitroglycerin tablets to sublingual spray, but it is likely that the onset of action following spray would be more rapid, and more reliable (the dissolution of sublingual tablets can be variable and affected my saliva volume) and the spray has greater long-term stability compared to tablets. Nonetheless, there is sufficient indirect evidence to suggest the beneficial role of prophylactic sublingual nitroglycerin therapy; and to suggest greater use for this approach.

References

[1] Aronow, W.S.: Drug therapy: Management of stable angina. N. Engl. J. Med. 289 (1973) 516–520.

[2] Chevigne, P., P. Colfignon, H. Kulbertus: Hemodynamic response to glyceryl trinitrate in a spray at rest and during exercise in a sitting position. Cardiology 69 (1982) 84–90.

[3] Chevigne, P., J. Renier, P. Rigo et al.: Efficaele de la nitroglycerine en nebuliseur. Revue Med. Interne 1 (1980) 265–272.

[4] Detry, J.M.R., R.A. Bruce: Effects of nitroglycerin on "maximal" oxygen intake and exercise electrocardiogram in coronary heart disease. Circulation 43 (1971) 155–163.

[5] Fanelli, C., R. Zelis, J.A. Gasscho: Comparison of venodilatory effects of nitroglycerin spray and tablets in healthy volunteers. Am. J. Cardiol. 63 (1989) 637–639.
[6] Feske, W., S.M. Finkelstein, G. Francis et al.: Vascular compliance after nitroprusside in hypertension. IEEE Proc. 14 (1988) 277–280.
[7] Gage, J.E., O.M. Hess et al.: Vasoconstriction of stenotic coronary arteries during dynamic exercise in patients with classic angina pectoris; Reversibility by nitroglycerin. Third Edition.
[8] Glasser, S.P., D.K. Arnett , G.E. McVeigh et al.: Vascular compliance and cardiovascular disease: A risk factor or a marker? Am. J. Hypertens. 10 (1997) 1175–1189.
[9] Glasser, S.P., D.K. Arnett , G.E. McVeigh et al.: The importance of arterial compliance in cardiovascular crug therapy. J. Clin. Pharmacol. 38 (1998) 202–212.
[10] Kimchi, A., G. Lee, E. Amsterdam et al.: Increased exercise tolerance after nitroglycerin oral spray:a new and effective therapeutic modality in angina pectoris. Circulation 67(l) (1983) 125–127.
[11] Naito, H., Y. Matsuda, K. Shiomi et al.: Effects of sublingual nitrate in patients receiving sustained therapy of isosorbide dinitrate for coronary artery disease. Am. J. Cardiol. 64 (1998) 565–568.
[12] Parker, J.O., K.A. Vankoughnet, B. Farrell: Nitroglycerin lingual spray: Clinical efficacy and dose-response relation. Am. J. Cardiol. 57 (1986) 1–5.
[13] Smulyan, H., M.D. Mookherjee, R.A. Warner: The effect of nitroglycerin on forearm arterial distensibility. Circulation 73 (1986) 1264–1269.
[14] Steering Committee, Transdermal Nitroglycerin Cooperative Study. Acute and chronic antianginal efficacy of continuous twenty-four-hour application of transdermal nitroglycerin. Am. J. Cardiol. 68 (1991) 1263–1273.
[15] Stipe, A.S., G.B. Fink: Prophylactic therapy of angina pectoris with organic nitrates: relationship of drug efficacy and clinical experimental design. J. Clin. Pharmacol. 13 (1973) 244–249.
[16] Thadani, U., R.J. Lipicky: Short and long-acting oral nitrates for stable angina pectoris. Cardiovasc. Drugs Ther. 8(6) (1991) 611–623.
[17] Thadani, U., J.O. Parker: Influence of glyceryl trinitrate during supine and upright exercise in patients with angina pectoris. Br. Heart J. 40 (1978) 1229–1236.

Psychological guidance of patients with coronary heart disease

W. Langosch

Development and maintenance of health-related behavior modification

Health education programs are the center piece of in-hospital cardiologic rehabilitation. Participation is mandatory for hospital patients with coronary heart disease and attendance is taken. Therefore, it can be assumed that patients are well-informed about the main risk factors and know what kind of changes are necessary to check on or attenuate further progression of coronary artery disease.

However, having the knowledge does not necessarily mean that patients are willing or able to transfer resolutions made in the hospital into everyday life outside the hospital. To achieve their goals they need active help from other persons that are important in their life. Primary or family physicians have a prominent role as they are the patient's personal expert on health matters and lifestyle changes for medical reasons.

Physicians can assume that their patients are interested in modifying their behavior; yet, it remains to be seen how strong their desire is and how serious their efforts are. Thus, it is useful and sensible to assess the individual's willingness to change according to the "stages of change" for behavior modification of Prochaska et al. [3, 9].

The authors distinguish five steps. Patients on the first stage are not interested in changing their behavior. It is assumed that patients after in-hospital treatment for coronary heart disease have at least reached the second stage, where behavior modification is taken into consideration, or even the third stage, where firm resolutions are being made. The two highest stages refer to active behavior change and maintenance of these changes. This division of the motivation to change behavior into different stages underlines that the decision to change one's lifestyle is a complex process and not a single, one-time event, and that, after the initial decision has been made, further measures are needed in order to achieve and maintain a behavior modification.

Allmer [1] constructed a model representing recent knowledge on development and maintenance of health-related behavior. According to this model, there is an initial development of an intention to act based on a subjective judgment process consisting mainly of two components:

1. the intensity of the desire to be healthy, i.e., the subjective evaluation of the importance of the intended lifestyle change for the patients health and
2. the patient's conviction that his own actions can lead to this desired state of health. This conviction is essential for the patient assuming responsibility for his or her own health.

Combination of these two components creates a kind of self-commitment to health-related activity for the patient, i.e., taking over personal responsibility for one's own health is the result of an individual evaluation of subjective importance and one's own ability to control the situation.

During the following phase of resolution formation patients think about ways of realizing their intentions. They ponder alternative ways to find the best course of action, i.e., the kind of behavior modification that promises to be most efficient compared with their effort.

The estimated effort is a calculation of what kind of effort will be necessary for various alternative courses of action. The estimate depends largely on the assessment of the individual abilities and if they are sufficient enough to change the behavior and whether the environment encourages or inhibits these changes.

The estimated effect balances negative and positive consequences that are attached to the different alternatives, and looks at the probability of these consequences to occur. Among the anticipated effects are emotional and/or psychosocial strains that can result from different actions. The estimated likelihood of a particular consequence to occur is related to an emotional evaluation including feelings such as trust, optimism, pessimism, and apprehension. The patient chooses the alternative promising the most efficient effort–effect ratio. Once a resolution to act has been made, the degree of self-commitment increases, i.e., the extent to which the patient feels bound to his resolution.

However, experience teaches us that not all resolutions are transmitted into concrete action, otherwise there would be no need for support from other persons or for favorable conditions. A precondition for realizing the resolution in concrete action is that the resolution can overcome

- situational obstructions, such as lack of social support,
- other current temptations,
- and competing interests.

Often realization is not abandoned immediately, but rather postponed, in order to avoid a feeling of guilt or disapproval from others. This gives the patient a chance to restart at a later date under the theme of "There's always another day that I can do something for my health."

Actual realization of health-related behavior is not possible without willpower. In order to act the way he wants to,

1. the patient has to be convinced that he can overcome the expected or real resistance
2. he also has to be able to protect his resolution from competing interests as well as from other current temptations.

Major components of willpower as far as health-related behavior is concerned, are self-initiative, determination, and perseverance. These components aid not only in the protection of health-related intentions from disturbing influences, but also in the performance and maintenance of these intentions regardless of anticipated or actual problems. In addition to willpower, an optimal basic motivation to perform the intended action is necessary. Excessive motivation is as unfavorable as a lack of motivation. Sign of an excessive basic motivation is, among others, a lack of calm and composure which makes it impossible to tolerate a temporary standstill or a setback in achieving the goal or to judge the action as a failure if the change of behavior within a certain period of time appears insufficient. A lack of basic motivation is marked by listlessness, lack of energy, and lack of drive.

Duits et al. [5] reported that patients with a lack of confidence and lack of symptoms prior to coronary artery disease have increased anxiety and depression scores 6 months after the events. According to the model suggested by Allmer [1], resolution formation as well as realization of necessary health-related changes in lifestyle have to work against increased difficulties in these patients with a myocardial infarction or coronary bypass operation, as they have a tendency to underestimate the positive effects of behavior changes and to overestimate the anticipated negative effects. Beyond that, one must assume:

1. they do not have the willpower they need to protect their resolution from disturbing influences and
2. they do not posses the basic motivation needed to maintain their resolution in the face of internal and external problems (e.g., boredom, lethargy, premature stop, dysphoria, lack of social support, unhealthy behavior of other persons at social functions).

Thus, these patients constitute a problem group that needs special support if the goal of a health-promoting change in lifestyle shall be achieved.

A model for health counseling by the family physician

An important precondition for execution and maintenance of health-related behavior in everyday life is the patient's acceptance of responsibility for his own health and his conviction that he can make the necessary changes by himself. Arborelius [2] suggests rules for health counseling by physicians that are designed to help the patient build up this conviction:

1. Describe the intended health behavior in as much detail as possible.
2. Quantify the current problem behavior, i.e., the unhealthy behavior, in order to counteract tendencies to play down the unhealthy consequences and in order to properly determine the extent of the necessary change in behavior.
3. Lead the patient to the decision whether or not to take on the effort of changing his behavior. The physician's task is, firstly, to provide the patient with all information needed to arrive at an estimate of the effort required for and the effect of the different alternatives and, secondly, to offer encouragement as well as actual help and support in order to motivate the patient to decide in favor of a health-promoting alternative. Arborelius especially emphasizes that the decision has to be the patient's own decision carried by his conviction that he wants to change his behavior, and not one made in order to please the physician or because he submits to the physician's authority.
4. Help the patient to change his behavior. Physicians can support a patient in resisting against competing temptations, can have a positive influence on his basic motivation, and can strengthen his willpower. These tasks are made easier if the patient is encouraged to record his target behavior, as this allows for a direct comparison of his achieved behavior changes with his goal.
5. Encourage and reinforce the patient's progress and achievements on his way towards his goal through appreciation and praise. However, make sure that the patient can accept this praise as being earned.

Arborelius [2] suggests the following agenda for health counseling:

1. Make clear why the patient's "change of lifestyle" is being addressed. The patient has to understand that the physician is not trying to promote a healthy lifestyle as a general measure but as a specific means of reducing the individual coronary risk.
2. Quantification of selected health-related behavior; while doing so, the physician should inquire about situational dependence, e.g., so-called temptation situations.
3. The direct connection of the patient's symptoms and his previous health-damaging behavior has to be worked out.

4. Finding out the patient's conviction as to which factors were responsible for his disease and could influence the future course of his disease.
   The physician's task is to determine the patient's causal attributions and control beliefs. A study by De Valle and Norman [4] showed a close connection of lifestyle change and causal attribution. The authors found that patients who had successfully changed their diet were also those who had most believed that wrong eating habits were a major cause of their disease.
5. In case the patient cannot decide to change his behavior, the physician should try to find out what makes the patients stick with his health-damaging behavior or what obstacles could be in the way of a behavior change. The following discussion of pros and cons of various target behaviors works out an effort-effect ratio for each alternative, thus motivating the patient to opt for a healthy lifestyle change.
6. Once the patient has made a decision in favor of a change in behavior, the primary aim is to ease execution of the change. First of all, one must agree upon a realistic and clear target behavior. Then the patient has to learn about techniques that will help him reach this target and, if necessary, these techniques should be rehearsed. Together, patient and physician have to identify internal and external conditions that could promote or inhibit the patient's efforts to achieve his goal.
7. The patient has to be prepared to cope with specific situational temptations. During the counseling the physician has to actively reinforce the patient's own belief that his efforts and his resolution will be efficacious.
8. During the execution period the patient should receive positive feedback about the changes in his behavior he has achieved. The defined behavior targets have to be adjusted to the real situation. The feedback should include recognition of the achieved approximation to the target. The feedback is much more effective if the verbal encouragement and confirmation is backed up with objective and quantitative data. If there are relapses, patient and physician should analyze the specific situation, trying to find positive consequences for the future and to develop strategies to avoid further relapses. It is of the utmost importance that a relapse does not cause the patient to give up on his goal or to give in to a feeling of powerlessness as the so-called breach of abstinence effect leads the patient to go back to his former unhealthy behavior or even to indulge in worse behavior patterns.

A study by Lovibond et al. [8] has shown that such extensive approaches produce the best results.

The main characteristics of this strategy, which was termed "maximum behavior modification" by the authors, are:

1. A behavior analysis to identify unhealthy behavior pattern as well as conditions favoring this wrong behavior.
2. Selection of realistic short and long term targets for behavior modification. As long term goals, e.g., ideal body weight, can be achieved only in the distant future, intermediate targets that can be reached within a reasonable period of time need to be defined.
3. Detailed information on behavior techniques which aid in achieving the short and long term goals.
4. Practicing a variety of self-management techniques that are designed to gain self-control over health-damaging behavior pattern. Correct application of the selected techniques was assessed regularly.
5. Repeated measurement of risk factors and regular feedback on the actual approximation to the target range, the actual individual risk, and the decrease in individual risk for coronary disease over the next five years. Discrepancies between diaries and objective data were discussed thoroughly.

Maximum behavior modification was divided into a two-month period of therapy and a four-month stabilization period. During the therapy period, patients attended weekly 90-minute counseling sessions, as well as biweekly sessions during the stabilization period. To increase the chances for success, the patient's partner was allowed to attend the counseling sessions and some 20 % took advantage of this offer.

The results show that maximum behavior modification achieved far better results than the other two models. Patients in this treatment group had the highest weight reduction during the six-month intervention period, as well as during the follow-up period of 12 months. On average, they lost 9.6 kg, whereas the other groups lost 8.3 kg and 5.5 kg respectively. Similar results were reported for systolic and diastolic blood pressure. At the end of the twelve-month follow-up period, daily nicotine consumption of smokers in the maximum treatment group was down by 64.4 %, while the other groups showed reductions of 29.4 % and 29 %.

The risk for the maximum treatment group to sustain a coronary event within the next 5 years dropped by 41 %, as opposed to only 35 % and 20 % for the other groups.

The authors suspect that maintenance of the positive effects throughout the follow-up period is partially due to the fact that the lifestyle changes were reinforced positively by "natural" side-effects such as increased well-being, increased satisfaction with one's general appearance, and an increased sense of self-effectiveness.

Recommendations for health counseling of patients with coronary heart disease by primary or family physicians

Based on the models and therapy approaches discussed here, the following recommendations for health counseling of patients with coronary heart disease by primary or family physicians can be made:

1. Patients showing signs of anxiety or depression need special attention, particularly those who show a lack of self-confidence and a tendency towards hypochondria.
2. To help the patient arrive at a positive effort and effect estimate, the physician has to explain the coronary risk associated with continuation of the current unhealthy lifestyle as well as the reduction in risk that can be achieved by adhering to a healthy lifestyle.
3. The counseling technique has to be patient-centered and the following techniques are advantageous as they encourage communication: clarification, explanation, checking of understanding, open questions, summarization, talking about and registration of feelings.
   Techniques that could impair communication have to be avoided: giving orders, rebukes, moralizing, offering solutions too quickly, impatience with pauses in the conversation, premature interpreting, depreciatory remarks, talking about oneself, overly empathic praise or criticism.

4. Only realistic short and medium term behavior targets that can be reached within a reasonable period of time should be agreed upon; unrealistically high or far-off targets should be avoided.
5. The behavior change has to be a therapeutic task for the patient [6], i.e., he has to know what to do and how often he is supposed to do it, how to record his behavior, what consequences achievement of the goal has as well as non-achievement, and that he has to bring his behavior record to the next session.
6. Potential situational temptations have to be addressed in advance to prepare the patient for these difficult situations. If relapses occur, the patient should be encouraged to continue with his program, and it should be pointed out that a temporary setback or occasional relapse does not constitute a definite failure.

One of the advantages of the office-based care of patients with coronary artery disease is that primary or family physicians can promote the behavior modification by prescribing drugs that increase the physical capacity of patients, thus increasing confidence in their own body while reducing their anxiety level and/or raising their spirit. Substances that allow patients to be more active physically and thereby exert a positive effect on their psychological make-up are an example for such agents.

The meta-analysis performed by Linden et al. [7] has shown additional psychosocial intervention reduces coronary risk factors as well as cardiac mortality significantly in patients with coronary artery disease. We can therefore assume that the best approach to improving the long-term prognosis for patients with coronary artery disease is treatment by family or primary physicians with a regimen combining drug therapy with goal-directed behavior modification towards a health-promoting lifestyle.

References

[1] Allmer, H.: Gesundheitsverhalten als intentionales und volitives Geschehen. In: Schwarzer, R. (Hrsg.): Gesundheitspsychologie, S. 117–130. Hogrefe, Göttingen 1992.

[2] Arborelius, E.: Using doctor-patient communication to affect patients' lifestyles. Theoretical and practical implications. Psychology and Health 11 (1996) 845–855.

[3] Basler, H.-D., S. Keller: Gesundheitsberatung. In: Gerber, W.-D., H.-D. Basler, U. Tewes (Hrsg.): Medizinische Psychologie, S. 383–389. Hogrefe, Göttingen 1994.

[4] De Valle, M.N., P. Norman: Causal attributions, health locus of control beliefs and lifestyle changes among pre-operative coronary patients. Psychology and Health 7 (1992) 201–211.

[5] Duits, A.A., H.J. Duivenvoorden, S. Boeke et al.: A structural modelling analysis of anxiety and depression in patients undergoing coronary artery bypass graft surgery: A modell generating approach. J. Psychosom. Res. 46 (1999) 187–200.

[6] Kanfer, F., H. Reinecker, D. Schmelzer: Selbst-Management-Therapie. Springer, Berlin 1996.

[7] Linden, W., C. Stossel, J. Maurice: Psychosocial interventions for patients with coronary artery disease. A meta-analysis. Archives Internal Med. 156 (1996) 745–752.

[8] Lovibond, S.H., P.C. Birell, P. Langeluddecke: Changing coronary heart disease risk-factor status: The effects of three behavioral programs. J. Behav. Med. 9 (1986) 415–437.

[9] Prochaska, J., C. DiClemente, M. Verdi: Understanding yourself as a smoker. Mancini, East Greenwich, Rhode Island 1987.

Hypertension therapy in patients with coronary heart disease

J. Scholze

Introduction

Hypertension and coronary heart disease can occur independent of each other. However, most of the time hypertension induces or accelerates arteriosclerotic processes that lead to coronary sclerosis and finally to coronary heart disease. This pathogenetic sequence involves monocytes in form of a proinflammatory reaction (increase of TNFα and IL-1-β under stimulation) and through increased adherence to the endothelium, as well as the endothelium itself through impaired dilative capacity (endothelial dysfunction [11]) (Fig. 1).

Based on the fact that arteriosclerotic processes can start early in life, it has been assumed that both genetics as well as the known classical risk factors play an important part and this model has been proven by the results of two large, long-term studies in the USA, the Bogalousa Heart Study and the Muscatine Study.

The Bogalousa Heart Study involved children and young adults who had been screened for risk factors of coronary heart disease since birth. With more than 5,000 children and young adults between the ages of 9 and 17 involved, it could be shown that known risk factors are present at a young age. In 1986 autopsy results from 35 children who had died – mostly in accidents – and whose risk factor constellation had been known were published [25]. There were clearly visible signs of lipid infiltration of vessel walls (aorta, coronaries) and the extent of these lesions could be correlated to the cholesterol levels and the arterial blood pressure. 12 years later, in 1998, data from more than 200 children and young men (aged 2 to 39) were available and these data

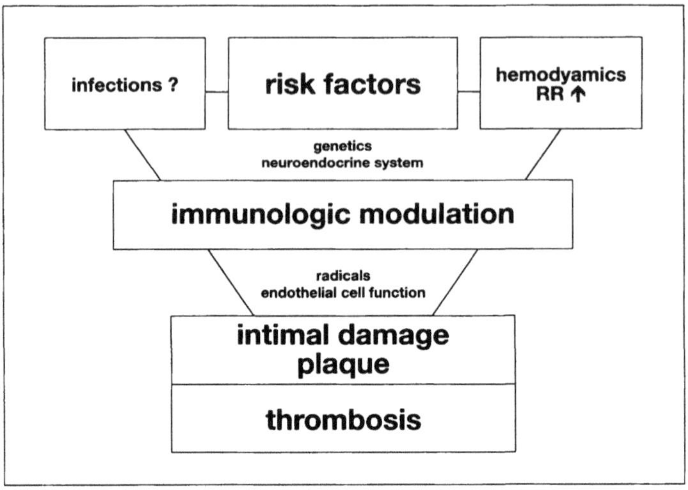

Fig. 1 Pathogenesis of thromboembolic events.

confirmed the initial findings [3]. These spectacular results show that all autopsied children and young adults already had fatty streaks in the aorta and that 50 % of children aged 2 to 15 showed these changes in the coronaries (as well as 85 % of participants aged 21–39). Fibrous plaques of the aorta were found in approximately 35 % of the 16–20 years group and in 50 % of the 21–25 years group. The extend of these early arteriosclerotic lesions correlated with arterial blood pressure, smoking, BMI, and cholesterol level (LDL, TG), and an accumulation of risk factors proved especially harmful. Similar data were received from the Pathological Determinants of Atherosclerosis in Youth (PDAY) study [37].

Apart from a great deal of data concerning accumulation of risks, the Bogalousa Heart Study also shows a marked increase in average body weight by some 0.2 kg (0.5 lb) per year over the last twenty years. In the Muscatine Study, one quarter of children and young adults aged 6–18 had elevated cholesterol levels and approximately one tenth of students aged 14 to 16 had high blood pressure [22, 28].

In conclusion, we can say these studies prove that arteriosclerotic changes start at an early age, take a slow progressive course, and mainly depend on the individual risk profile of patients, in children as well as young adults and later on in life. Whether or not chlamydial infection or other infections play a relevant part in this process cannot be answered at this point in time.

New classification of hypertension and target values for blood pressure

As there is no doubt about the importance of elevated blood pressure or hypertension, respectively, for the induction and progression of arteriosclerotic processes, especially those involving the coronaries, keeping the blood pressure within a strictly set normal range has to be a therapeutic goal.

Until 1998 there was considerable uncertainty, primarily due to the results of the retrospective case-control study of Cruickshank [7] on the effects of lowering of blood pressure, and a J-shaped relation of blood pressure and coronary mortality was discussed, but the results of the prospective, randomized HOT study [17] refuted this hypothesis. This study, which involved more than 19,000 patients, did not show an increase in coronary morbidity or mortality for blood pressure lower than 85 mmHg in patients with hypertension and without accompanying illness. It also did not show an increase in patients with hypertension and coronary heart disease and/or diabetes mellitus. It was even shown that the prognosis of high-risk patients in particular improved under an intensive lowering of blood pressure to values of 82 mmHg or even lower.

Based on these unmistakable results, which are in line with the results of the UKPD study of diabetics (significant reduction in mortality of type II diabetics with intensive blood pressure lowering 144/82 vs. 154/87: stroke reduced by 44 %, heart failure by 56 % [40, 41]) WHO and ISH (International Society on Hypertension) reacted quickly and redefined their classification of hypertension, adjusting it to the American point of view (Tab. 1). One should note the definition of a high-normal range, which will trigger the onset of therapy in high-risk patients, and the clear-cut definition of hypertension from 140/90 mmHG

Table 1 Definitions and classification of blood pressure levels [15]

category	systolic [mmHg]	diastolic [mmHg]
optimal	< 120	< 80
normal	< 130	< 85
high-normal	130–139	85–89
hypertension		
grade 1 (mild)	140–159	90–99
subgroup: borderline	140–149	90–94
grade 2 (moderate)	160–179	100–109
grade 3 (severe)	≥ 180	≥ 110
isolated systolic hypertension	≥ 140	< 90
subgroup: borderline	140–149	< 90

upwards, regardless of age, sex or other factors [15, 19]. The individual assignment of cardiovascular risk scores to patients with hypertension is based on risk factors, damage to end-organs, and associated relevant factors (Tab. 2).

Using the same premises, the target ranges for blood pressure was up-dated (Tab. 3).

Pathophysiologic connection between hypertension and (coronary) arteriosclerosis

From a pathophysiologic point of view, arteriosclerotic processes are complex as well.

Apart from hemodynamic factors (shearing forces, pulsations, and so forth) neuroendocrinologically triggered mechanisms are of importance (Figs. 1

Table 2 Cardiovascular risk stratification of patients with hypertension based on risk factors, target-organ damage and associated clinical conditions [15]

Risk factors for cardiovascular diseases

- levels of systolic and diastolic blood pressure
- men age > 55 years
- women age > 65 years
- smoking
- total cholesterol > 6.5 mmol/l (250 mg/dl)
- diabetes
- family history of premature cardiovascular disease

Target-organ damage

- left ventricular hypertrophy (electrocardiogram, echocardiogram)
- proteinuria and/or elevated plasma creatinine (1.2–2.0 mg/dl)
- ultrasound or radiological evidence of arteriosclerotic plaques (carotid, iliac and femoral arteries, aorta)

Associated clinical conditions

- cerebrovascular disease
  ischemic stroke
  cerebral hemorrhage
  transient ischemic attack
- heart disease
  myocardial infarction
  angina pectoris
  coronary revascularization
  congestive heart failure
- renal disease
  diabetic nephropathy
  renal failure (creatinine > 2.0 mg/dl)
- vascular disease
  dissecting aneurysm
  symptomatic arterial disease
- severe hypertensive retinopathy
  haemorrhages, exsudates
- papilloedema

Table 3 Target blood pressure values [15, 19]

a)	general, elderly patients	< 140/90 mmHg
	younger and middle aged patients	< 130/85 mmHg
	ambulatory blood pressure monitoring	< 135/85 mmHg
b)	severe associated clinical conditions	
	diabetes mellitus congestive heart failure renal failure	< 130/85 mmHg ideal 125/80 mmHg

and 2). Endothelial dysfunction occupies center stage not only as an effector organ, but also as mediator of subsequent proliferation and adhesion and procoagulatory processes. We know from exact studies by the American working group of J. Laragh and M. H. Alderman [2] that patients with high renin levels have an increased risk of suffering a myocardial infarction, regardless of their individual risk factor status. The sympathetic nervous system also plays a part not only in the development of chronic sclerotic processes but also in acute complications (Fig. 3) [20].

Differential drug therapy of hypertension in coronary heart disease

Evidence based data confirm a decrease of coronary mortality in the range of 10–14% when essential hypertension is treated with diuretics and beta-adrenergic blocking agents [6]. For older patients these figures are even better [39], apart from therapy with beta-adrenergic blocking agents [24], but all data concerning morbidity and mortality are worse than the results for the prevention of stroke (a reduction of approx. 40–45%). Insufficient lowering of blood pressure and intervention time, as well as neuroendocrine activation under diuretics and a lack of metabolic indifference have been discussed as reasons for these findings.

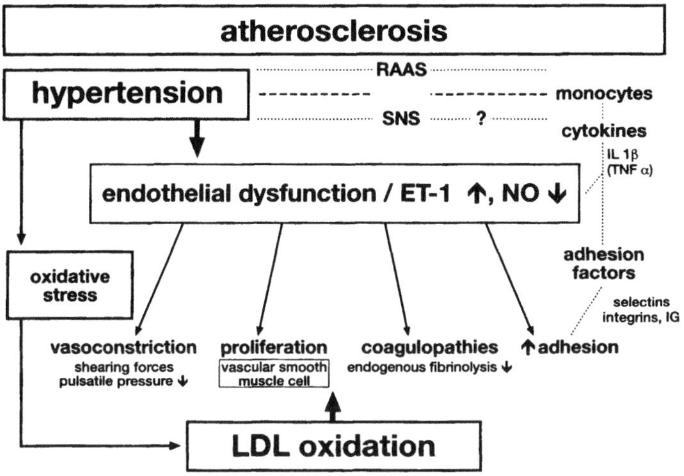

Fig. 2 Pathomechanisms of hypertension and atherosclerosis.

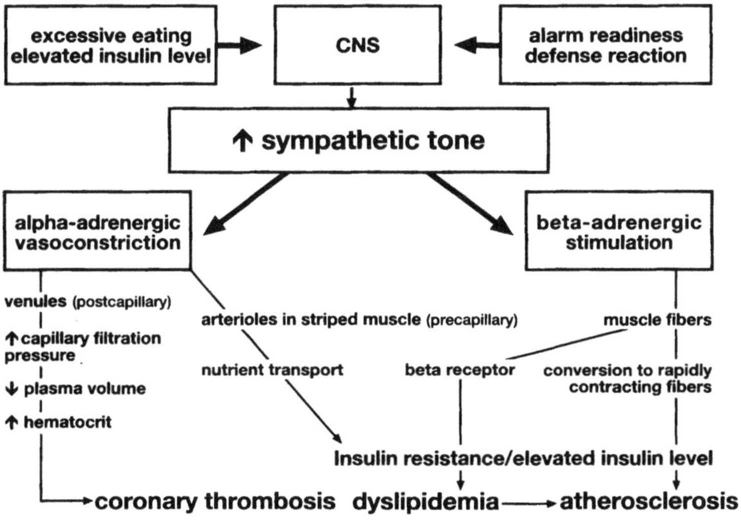

Fig. 3 Effects of an increased activity of the sympathetic nervous system on metabolism, atherosclerosis and coronary thrombosis.
(modified after Julius [20]).

Recent studies with calcium channel blockers (Syst-Eur study for systolic hypertension [36]) and ACE inhibitors (CAPPP study [16]) showed better results, especially in obvious high-risk patients with diabetes mellitus [16, 17].

The therapy guidelines of WHO/ISH and JNC VI recommend the use of beta-adrenergic blocking agents and calcium channel blockers for the treatment of angina in hypertension [15, 19].

A survey by the representatives of the German Hypertension League (Deutsche Hochdruckliga) showed that, apart from these substances, ACE inhibitors, AT_1-antagonists, and post-synaptic alpha-blockers are used regularly [30] (Tab. 4).

Beta-adrenergic blocking agents

The data concerning the use of beta-adrenergic blocking agents in primary prevention of coronary heart disease are less convincing and do not justify their preferred use. Especially in elderly patients, beta-adrenergic blocking agents are less effective than diuretics as far as coronary morbidity, cardiovascular mortality, and total mortality is concerned [24].

However, their use in secondary prevention after myocardial infarction has a proven track record with reduced rates of reinfarction (minus 27 %), sudden death (minus 22 %), and total mortality (minus 22 %) [43].

A reduced heart rate and cardiac workload not only decreases the cardiac oxygen consumption, but also increases myocardial perfusion time via a prolonged diastole and inhibits deleterious sympathetic effects that could cause rhythm disorders. All beta-blocking drugs, apart from beta-blocking agents with intrinsic sympathicomimetic activity, show these positive effects on morbidity and mortality; cardioselective substances are usually preferred, as they show less metabolic and pulmonary interactions. Vasodilating third generation beta-blocking agents have obvious advantages as far as hemodynamic aspects are concerned, there are, however, no data available concerning the long-term prognosis.

Table 4 Differential therapy of hypertension with associated illnesses. Evaluation of indication priorities for different substance groups (1: exceptionally efficacious ... to 4: not suitable or contraindicated) by an expert committee (Landesvertreter der deutschen Hochdruckliga) [30]

Differential drug therapy Evaluation by expert committee	diuretics	loop diuretics	β-blocking agents β-1-selective	non-selective	Ca-channel-blocker verapamil-type	dihydripyridine-type	ACE-inhibitors	postsynaptic α-blocking agent	antisympathotonics sympatholytic agents	direct vasodilators	AT_1-antagonists	moxonidine	fixed-combinations
Aspect: hypertension and left ventricular hypertrophy or coronary heart disease													
left ventricular hypertrophy	2.0	2.5	1.3	2.3	1.4	1.9	1.0	1.8	1.8	2.9	1.1	1.8	1.6
stable angina pectoris (AP)	1.9	1.9	1.0	2.0	1.3	2.5	1.3	1.8	2.0	3.0	1.4	2.0	1.6
unstable AP	2.0	2.1	1.1	2.3	1.5	3.4	1.5	2.1	2.1	3.2	1.5	2.5	2.2
acute myocardial infarction (MI)	2.0	2.0	1.2	2.0	2.0	3.6	1.5	2.2	2.4	3.4	1.7	2.5	3.0
long-term treatment after MI	1.8	2.1	1.1	2.0	1.4	3.0	1.1	2.0	2.1	3.0	1.4	2.1	1.9

Calcium antagonists

Based on existing experimental, pathophysiologic, and clinical (surrogate) data an anti-atherosclerotic efficacy of calcium antagonists seems apparent (Tab. 5). However, more than any other group of anti-hypertensive principles, calcium channel blockers have a great heterogeneity with variable points of action, different involvement of neuroendocrine systems. Thus they do have varying indications and show different clinical efficacy (Fig. 4) [31]. Verapamil (diltiazem) reduces heart rate and noradrenaline level significantly, whereas dihydropyridines have a contrary effect; yet, long-acting highly vasoselective dihydropyridine calcium antagonists do not pose the same problems as short-acting do and are still considered a safe option for treatment of high blood pressure and stable angina pectoris. A useful criterion for the selection of a substance is the initial heart rate, which can be seen as a rough measure for the sympathetic activity and thus for the cardiovascular status. Based on the heart rate data from the Framingham study [14] and its link with the long-term prognosis, we recommend the application of rate-lowering agents, such as verapamil, for average rates of higher than 80 beats per minute. In the APSIS-Study, verapamil achieved identical results as metoprolol as far as morbidity and mortality is concerned [27]. Especially the DAVIT-II-Study

Table 5 Anti-arteriosclerotic efficacy of calcium channel blockers – positive and negative effects

positive	*negative*
sNS activity ↓	sNS ↑ } DHP*
ET_1 induced vasoconstriction ↓	Angiotensin II ↑ } DHP*
antiproliferative potential	
interactions endothelium/VSMC/monocytes, platelets	
antithrombotic	
metabolically neutral	
antioxidative	
	*short-acting > long-acting

(DHP: dihydropyridine type calcium antagonists; ET_1: endothelin 1; sNS: sympathetic nervous system; VSMC: vascular smooth muscle cells)

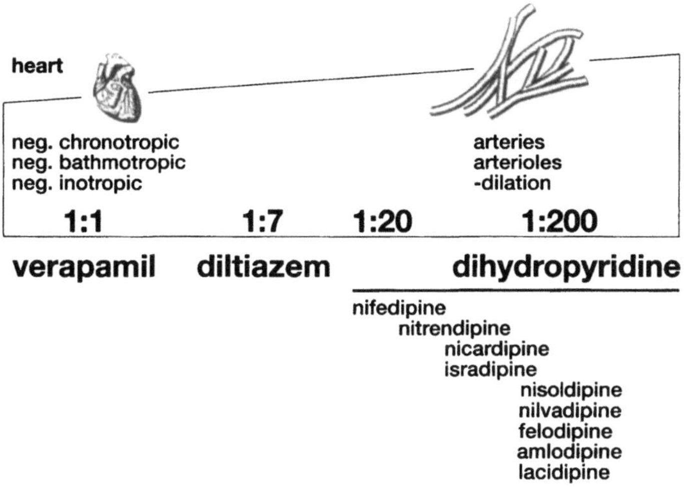

Fig. 4 Differentiation of calcium channel blockers based on heart/vessel selectivity ratio.

Table 6 Comparison of indications of verapamil and beta-blocking agents for clinical entities

verapamil has similar effects on circulation as selective beta-adrenergic blockers • HR, rhythm (negative chronotropic)
verapamil is superior to beta-adrenergic blockers • in vasodilation = lowering of diastolic blood pressure, PVD (exemption: vasodilating beta-blockers) • in patients with metabolic RF, chronic obstructive lung diseases
verapamil is inferior to beta-adrenergic blockers • ventricular arrhythmia • congestive heart failure (negative inotropism)

(PVD: peripheral vascular disease; HR: heart rate; RF: risk factors)

showed that verapamil is a true alternative to beta-adrenergic blocking agents in MI patients without heart failure and that it improves cardiovascular morbidity and mortality considerably [8]. This effect is even more pronounced in combination therapy with trandolapril [12]. Table 6 compares some clinical aspects of verapamil and beta-blocking agents.

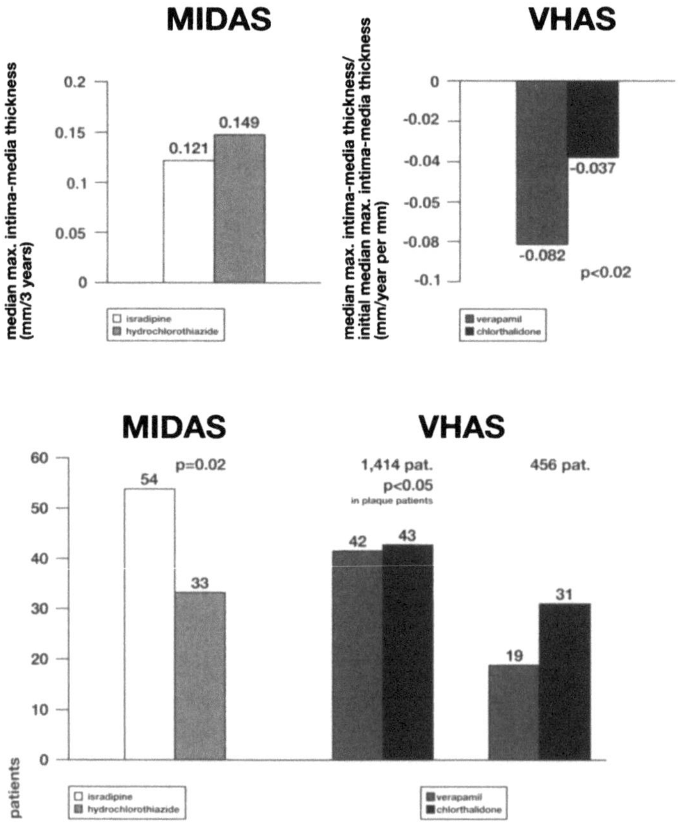

Fig. 5 Comparison of MIDAS- and VHAS-studies.
a) ultrasound findings carotid artery = primary endpoint
b) cardiovascular events
[1, 4, 44].

All studies published so far on dihydropyridine calcium channel blockers and arterial/coronary sclerosis (Intact [23], Montreal Heart [42], heart transplantation [35]) showed a reduced formation of new plaques without regression of already existing lesions. Two ultrasound studies on the course of carotid wall lesions reported differing results – no regression of intima-media thickness with isradipine (MIDAS); however, significantly better results for verapamil. Whereas the cardiovascular event rate was higher with isradipine than with HCT, the rate was lower for verapamil in patients with pre-existing plaques of the carotid artery in comparison to chlorthalidone (Fig. 5) [1, 4, 44]. Undecided is whether the increase in cardiovascular event rate with isradipine is due to the difference in blood pressure (more than 3 mm in favor of the calcium channel blocker) or triggered by the agent itself. Currently studies assessing the effects of third generation dihydropyridine type calcium channel blocker (lacidipine and amlodipine) on arteriosclerotic processes are in progress (ELSA study [45], PREVENT study).

It should be pointed out that only dihydropyridine type calcium channel blocker are contraindicated in unstable angina pectoris and myocardial infarction and that verapamil (diltiazem), when used in patients without heart failure, has improved prognosis (Tab. 7).

Table 7 Recommendations of the Board of the German Hypertension League (Deutsche Liga zur Bekämpfung des hohen Blutdrucks) for antihypertensive therapy with calcium channel blockers (shortened version May 1999)

1. Short-acting dihydropyridine type calcium channel blockers should not be used anymore.
2. In non-diabetic patients the usefulness of long-acting calcium antagonists is comparable to diuretics. This applies particulary to older patients with (isolated) systolic hypertension.
3. In patients with diabetes mellitus long-acting monotherapy with calcium antagonists appear to be superior to diuretics, but they are inferior to ACE inhibitors. Thus ACE inhibitors should be the drug of first choice. In diabetes mellitus a combination ACE inhibitor-calcium channel blocker is appropriate.
4. Dihydropyridines are contraindicated in patients with coronary heart disease and unstable angina pectoris, and myocardial infarction.

ACE inhibitors

The antiproliferative effects of ACE inhibitors, they improve endothelial dysfunction and inhibit the neuroendocrine system, make them a good choice for treatment of hypertension with coronary heart disease [32]. Apart from possessing NO-liberating effects, in combination with nitrates they inhibit nitrate tolerance.

So far only the CAPPP study has shown that ACE inhibitors have a positive influence on the reduction of coronary events in hypertension especially with diabetes mellitus [16]. Its benefit for secondary prevention (remodeling, reinfarction, heart failure, cardiovascular and total mortality) after myocardial infarction, however, has been proven impressively in a number of studies (SAVE, AIRE, TRACE and others [13, 21, 26, 38]).

Under aspects such as compliance and efficacy, and in order to achieve 24-hour cover, especially in the early morning hours, hypertension with accompanying coronary heart disease should only be treated with long-acting preparations with known 24-hour efficacy (Tab. 8) [18].

Platelet aggregation inhibitors

The HOT study showed for the first time that additional application of acetylsalicylic acid (ASS) (75 mg/day) was beneficial in the primary prevention of hypertension. ASS used by patients with well balanced antihypertensive medication reduced the number of myocardial infarctions, as well as the incidence of severe cardiovascular events without changing the stroke incidence [17]. Due to outstanding results in a number of studies, acetylsalicylic acid is an integral part of secondary prevention [29], yet, in Europe some 20% of patients with MI do not receive ASS [10]. When ASS is contraindicated, ticlopidine and clopidogrel are used for secondary prevention [5].

Table 8 Evaluating comparison of all ACE inhibitor currently approved in Europe [18]

Criteria	
through: peak ratio	1. trandolapril 2. ramipril/enalapril/cilazapril
efficacy	same for all agents
side-effects	same for all agents
variability in bioavailability	1. trandolapril
quality of life	1. AT_1 antagonists 2. ACE inhibitors
costs	depending on the country

Antihypertensive combination therapy

The HOT as well as the UKPD study showed that, in order to achieve normal blood pressure values, one half to three quarters of patients require combination therapy. This, of course, applies to our patients as well, at least as far as normotonia is concerned. In hypertension with coronary heart disease (angina pectoris) as concomitant disorder two primary treatment options can be distinguished:

beta-adrenergic blocking agents as basis therapy
 i.e., beta-adrenergic blocking agents plus dihydropyridine calcium antagonists
 or ACE inhibitors (AT_1 blockers)
initial therapy with verapamil
 i.e., sustained release verapamil plus ACE inhibitor (AT_1 blocker) (e.g. Udramil™ [in Germany: Verapamil SR/trandolapril]).

If more substances are required for a triple therapy diuretics, long-acting nitrates (in sufficient doses for patients with symptomatic angina pectoris, e.g. Monopur® ret. 60 once in the morning) or post-synaptic α-receptor blocking agents can be used.

Whenever possible, one should try using fixed combinations to reduce the number of tablets or pills patients have to take, as this helps increase compliance and is more economical. The main combinations with exceptional efficacy and compatibility are beta-blocking agent plus dihydropyridine type calcium antagonist and verapamil SR plus trandolapril [34]. The combination of verapamil SR plus trandolapril (Udramil™) fulfills all requirements of a good combination therapy, i.e., addition of therapeutic effects and low dosage for the individual agents, compensation of side-effects, and synergistic action on target organs (Tab. 9).

Table 9 Characteristics of the combination trandolapril plus verapamil (e.g. Udramil™)

• reliable efficacy	antihypertensive/antianginal
• cardioprotective	heart-rate-lowering 0_2-consumption ↓ coronary-dilating endothelial function ↑ (angiogenesis) length of diastole ↑ 0_2-supply ↑
• nephroprotective	microalbuminuria ↓, proteinuria ↓
• metabolically indifferent	cholesterol, triglyceride, glucose, uric acid
• neuroendocrine activity ↓	sympathetic tone ↓ RAAS ↓

References

[1] Agabiti-Rosei, E., C. Dal Palú, G. Leonetti et al. on behalf of the VHAS Investigators: Clinical results of the verapamil in hypertension and atherosclerosis study. J. Hypert. 15 (1997) 1337–1344.

[2] Alderman M.H., S. Madhavan, W.L. Ooi et al.: Association of the renin-sodium profile with the risk of myocardial infarction in patients with hypertension. N. Engl. J. Med. 324 (1991) 1098–1104.

[3] Berenson G.S., S.R. Srinivasan, W. Bal et al.: Association between multiple cardiovascular risk factors and atherosclerosis in children and young adults. The Bogalousa Heart Study. N. Engl. J. Med. 4 (1998) 338 (23) 1650–1656.

[4] Borhani, N.O., M. Mercuri, P.A. Borhani et al.: Final outcome results of the Multi-center Isradipine Diuretic Atherosclerosis Study (MIDAS). A randomized controlled trial. JAMA 276 (1996) 785–791.

[5] Christ, M., H.C. Diener, T. Kurth et al.: Sekundärprävention atherosklerotischer Erkrankungen in der täglichen Praxis. Internist 39 (1998) 1080–1097.

[6] Collins, R., R. Peto, S. MacMahon et al.: Blood pressure, stroke, and coronary heart diesease. Part 2, short-term reductions in blood pressure: overview of randomised drug trials in their epidemiological context. Lancet 335 (1990) 827–839.

[7] Cruickshank, J.M., J.M Thorp, F.J. Zacharias: Benefits and potential harm of lowering high blood pressure. Lancet I (1987) 581–583.

[8] Danish Study Group on Verapamil in Myocardial Infarction: Effect of verapamil on mortality and major events after acute myocardial infarction [The Danish Verapamil Infarction Trial II (DAVIT II)]. Am. J. Cardiol. 66 (1990) 779–785.

[9] Doerffel, Y., C. Lätsch, G. Burmester et al.: Activated Peripheral Monocytes in Essential Hypertension. Hypert. (1999).

[10] Euroaspire Group: A European Society of Cardiology survey of secondary prevention of coronary heart disease. Eur. Heart J. 18 (1997) 1569–1582.

[11] Ferro, J.Ch., D.F. Webb: Endothelial Dysfunction and Hypertension. Drugs 53, Suppl. 1 (1997) 30–41.

[12] Fischer Hansen, J., L. Hagerup, B. Sigurd et al. for the Danish Verapamil Infarction Trial (DAVIT) Study Group: Cardiac event rates after acute myocardial infarction in patients treated with verapamil and trandolapril versus trandolapril alone. Am. J. Cardiol. 79 (1997) 738–741.

[13] Garg, R., S. Yusuf for the Collaborative Group on ACE Inhibitor Trials: Overview of randomized trials of angiotensin-converting enzyme inhibitors on mortality and morbidity in patients with heart failure. JAMA 273 (1995) 1450–1456.

[14] Gillman, M.W., W.B. Kannel, A. Belanger et al.: Influence of heart rate on mortality among persons with hypertension: The Framingham Study. Am. Heart J. 125 (1993) 1148–1154.

[15] Guidelines Subcommittee: 1999 World Health Organization – International Society of Hypertension Guidelines for the Management of Hypertension. J. Hypert. 17 (1999) 151–183.

[16] Hansson, L., L.H. Lindholm, L. Niskanen et al.: Effect of angiotensin-converting-enzyme inhibition compared with conventional therapy on cardiovascular morbidity and mortality in hypertension: the Captopril Prevention Project (CAPPP) randomised trial. Lancet 353 (1999) 611–616.

[17] Hansson, L., A. Zanchetti, S.G. Carruthers et al. for the HOT Study Group: Effects of intensive blood pressure lowering and low-dose aspirin in patients with hypertension: principal results of the Hypertension Optimal Treatment (HOT) randomised trial. Lancet 351 (1998) 1755–1762.

[18] Janknegt, R., B.A.M. van Schalk, J. Smits et al.: ACE inhibitors and angiotensin II antagonists for the treatment of hypertension: Drug selection by means of the soja method. Eur. Hosp. Pharmacy 3 (1997) 46–58.

[19] Joint National Committee on Detection, Evaluation, and Treatment of High Blood Pressure. The sixth report of the Joint National Committee on Prevention, Detection, and Treatment of High Blood Pressure (JNC VI). Arch. Intern. Med. 157 (1997) 2413–2446.

[20] Julius, S.: Sympathetic hyperactivity and coronary risk in hypertension. Hypertension 21 (1993) 886–893.

[21] Kober, L., C. Torp-Pedersen, J.E. Carlsen et al.: A clinical trial of the angiotensin-converting-enzyme inhibitor trandolapril in patients with left ventricular dysfunction after myocardial infarction. Trandolapril Cardiac Evaluation (TRACE) Study Group. N. Engl. J. Med. 333 (1995) 1670–1676.

[22] Lauer, R.M., J. Lee, W.R. Clarke: Factors affecting the relationship between childhood and adult cholesterol levels: The Muscatine Study. Pediatrics 82 (1988) 309–318.

[23] Lichtlen, P.R., P.G. Hugenholtz, W. Rafflenbeul et al.: Retardation of angiographic progression of coronary artery disease by nifedipine. Lancet 335 (1990) 1109–1113.

[24] Messerli, F.H., E. Grossman, U. Goldbourt: Are beta-blockers efficacious as first-line therapy for hypertension in the elderly? A systematic review. JAMA 279 (1998) 1903–1907.

[25] Newmann, W.P., D.S. Freedmann, A.W. Voors et al.: Relation of serum lipoprotein levels an systolic blood pressure to early atherosclerosis. The Bogalousa Heart Study. N. Engl. J. Med. 17 314 (3) 183–144.

[26] Pfeffer, M.A., E. Braunwald, L.A. Moye et al.: Effect of captopril on mortality and morbidity in patients with left ventricular dysfunction after myocardial infarction. Results of the survival and ventricular enlargement trial. The SAVE Investigators. N. Engl. J. Med. 327 (1992) 669–677.
[27] Rehnquist, N., P. Hjemdahl, E. Billing et al.: Effects of metoprolol vs verapamil in patients with stable angina pectoris. Eur. Heart J. 17 (1996) 76–81.
[28] Rocchini, A.P., J. Key, D. Bondie et al: The effect of weight loss on the sensitivity of blood pressure to sodium in obsese adolescents. N. Engl. J. Med. 321 (1989) 580–585.
[29] Ryan, T.J., J.L. Anderson, E.M. Antman et al.: ACC/AHA guidelines for the management of patients with acute myocardial infarction. A report of the American College of Cardiology/American Heart Association Task Force on Practice Guidelines (Committee on Management of Acute Myocardial Infarction). J. Am. Coll. Cardiol. 28 (1996) 1328–1428.
[30] Scholze, J.: Hypertonie, Risikokonstellationen und Begleitkrankheiten, S. 630–631, 2. Aufl., Blackwell, Berlin-Wien 1999.
[31] Scholze, J.: Kalziumantagonisten. In: Scholze, J. (Hrsg): Hypertonie, Risikokonstellationen und Begleitkrankheiten, S. 80–92, 2. Aufl., Blackwell, Berlin-Wien 1999.
[32] Scholze, J.: ACE-Hemmstoffe. In: Scholze, J. (Hrsg): Hypertonie, Risikokonstellationen und Begleitkrankheiten, S. 93–119, 2. Aufl., Blackwell, Berlin-Wien 1999.
[33] Scholze, J.: Bluthochdruck und sympathisches Nervensystem: Einfluß der Herzfrequenz auf die Prognose. Herz Kreisl. 31 (1999) 247–253.
[34] Scholze, J., P. Zilles, D. Compagnone: Verapamil SR and trandolapril combination therapy in hypertension – a clinical trial of factorial design. Br. J. Clin. Pharmacol. 45 (5) (1998) 491–495.
[35] Schroeder, J.S., S.Z. Gao, E.L. Alderman et al.: A preliminary study of diltiazem in the prevention of coronary artery disease in heart transplant recipients. N. Engl. J. Med. 328 (1993) 164–170.
[36] Staessen, J.A., R. Fagard, L. Thijs et al. for the Systolic Hypertension in Europe (Syst-Eur) Trial Investigators: Randomised double-blind comparison of placebo and active treatment for older patients with isolated systolic hypertension. Lancet 350 (1997) 757–764.
[37] Strong, P., G.T. Malcom, M.C. Oalmann: Enviromental and genetic risk factors in early human atherogenesics: Lessons from the PADY study. Pathol. Intern. 45 (1995) 403–408.
[38] The Acute Infarction Ramipril Efficacy (AIRE) Study Investigators: Effect of ramipril on mortality and morbidity of survivors of acute myocardial infarction with clinical evidence of heart failure. Lancet 342 (1993) 821–828.

[39] Trenckwalder, P.: Hochdruck im fortgeschrittenen Lebensalter. In: Scholze, J. (Hrsg): Hypertonie, Risikokonstellationen und Begleitkrankheiten, S. 248–267, 2. Aufl., Blackwell, Berlin-Wien 1999.
[40] UK Prospective Diabetes Study Group. Tight blood pressure control and risk of macrovascular complications in type 2 diabetes: UKPDS 38. BMJ 317 (1998) 703–713.
[41] UK Prospective Diabetes Study Group. Efficacy of atenolol and captopril in reducing risk of macrovascular and microcascular complications in type 2 diabetes: UKPDS 39. BMJ 317 (1998) 713–720.
[42] Waters, D., J. Lesperance, M. Francetich et al.: A controlled trial to assess the effect of a calcium channel blocker on the progression of coronary atherosclerosis. Circulation 82 (1990) 1940–1953.
[43] Yusuf, S., R. Peto, J. Lewis et al.: Beta blockade during and after myocardial infarction: an overview of the randomized trials. Prog. Cardiovasc. Dis. 27 (1985) 335–371.
[44] Zanchetti, A., E. Agabiti-Rosei, C. Dal Palú for the VHAS Investigators: The Verapamil in Hypertension and Atherosclerosis Study (VHAS): results of long-term randomised treatment with either verapamil or chlorthalidone on carotis intima-media thickness. J. Hypertens. 16 (1998) 1667–1676.
[45] Zanchetti, A., M.G. Bond, M. Henning et al. on behalf of the ELSA Investigators: Risk factors associated with alterations in carotid intima-media thickness in hypertension: baseline data from the European Lacidipine Study on Atherosclerosis. J. Hypertens. 16 (1998) 949–961.

Awarding of the 1999 Nitrolingual Prize

Marianne Boskamp, Managing Director of the well-known pharmaceutical company Pohl-Boskamp awarded the Nitrolingual Prize to **Dr. Martina M. Brückmann** for her work **"Inducible NO synthase in smooth muscular cells – characterization and functional importance"**. The following offers a summary of the award-winning article and the announcement for the 2003 Nitrolingual Prize.

Subject of this paper is a comparison between undifferentiated ("pup cells") and highly-differentiated smooth muscle cells ("adult cells") in respect to their ability to express inducible NO synthase and to synthesize biologically active NO. Undifferentiated smooth muscle cells are found in abundance in the vascular media of neonatal animals. In the vessel walls of adult animals these cells are still present, although in rather low numbers, and they can increase in number under pathological conditions in order to aid in restoration of vessel wall lesions.

Analysis of nitrite (a stable oxidation product of NO) concentrations in the fluid above the cell sediment showed concentration-dependent and time-dependent release of nitrite from pup cells and adult cells after stimulation with the cytokines interleukin-1 β (IL-1 β) and tumor necrosis factor-α (TNF-α) as well as after treatment with lipopolysaccharide (LPS). IL-1 β-induced nitrite release was inhibited by the competitive NO synthase-inhibitor nitro L-arginine and totally blocked by the protein synthesis inhibitor cycloheximide. This points at expression of an inducible NO synthase. With the help of a specific antibody to inducible NO synthase of smooth vascular muscle cells it was possible to demonstrate that adult cells as well as pup cells are able to express a NO synthase of the inducible type after stimulation with cytokines. As adult cells release more nitrite and NO respectively, and synthesize more iNOS protein than pup cells, it can be assumed that NO synthase of adult cells is more easily induced than the one in pup cells.

The cell effluent of cytokine-stimulated adult and pup cells had a relaxing effect on vascular rings of the detector. This effect was traced back to the formation of biologically-active NO (or a NO-type compound) by the iNOS of adult and pup cells.

Electrophoretic mobility shift assays (EMSA) detected the occurrence of the transcription factor NF-κB in the cell nucleus after treatment of pup and adult cells with IL-1 β. This points at the involvement of NF-κB in cytokine-stimulated iNOS expression.

Expression of inducible NO synthase of adult and pup cells can be increased by growth factors and free components of the plasma (e.g. basic fibroblast growth factor and epidermal growth factor) as well as inhibited (e.g. transforming growth factor-β). However, the regulation mechanisms of iNOS expression are different in pup cells and adult cells.

Further experiments focused on the question whether the growth of cells with fetal properties is influenced by other means than the growth of highly-differentiated cells. Cell counts over a period of seven days showed a significantly higher proliferation rate of pup cells than of adult cells. The cytokine IL-β had a growth-inhibiting effect on pup cells but not on adult cells. Presence of different NO donators (furoxans and sodium nitroprusside) caused a proliferation inhibition of both pup cells and adult cells, an effect most likely due to release of NO or some NO metabolite. Antiproliferative effects of NO donators were more pronounced in adult cells than pup cells.

This study shows under pathological conditions mechanisms that already played a role in the development of the vessel wall (e.g. ability to proliferate) can become important again. Therapeutic procedures (e.g. medical prevention or treatment of restenosis after balloon angioplasty) have to take these special conditions into consideration: Therapeutic application of NO donators is probably an efficient way of inhibiting the proliferation of muscle cells in the vicinity of vascular lesions. NO donators with a low level release of NO over an extended period of time are most efficient. 3,4-subsituted furoxans could be suitable for in vivo prevention of restenosis after balloon dilatation of vessels as they have such a release profile and because there are no signs for tolerance formation for these substances.

Announcement “2003 Nitrolingual Prize”

In order to promote the medical research Pohl-Boskamp has initiated the “Hamburg Nitroglycerin Symposia” as well as the Nitrolingual Prize inviting entries for a competition for the first time in 1977.

The Nitrolingual Prize will be awarded to one study on new clinical and pharmacological novelties in the therapy with nitroglycerin. The themes are not only limited to the known sublingual and parenteral applications of nitroglycerin with the indication “coronary insufficiency”; of special interest are also the peroral, percutaneous, rectal and other forms of association with further indications such as cor pulmonale, peripheral circulatory disorders, acute pancreatitis, diseases of the biliary ducts, hypertensive crisis, sudden loss of hearing and other theoretical questions regarding the effects of nitroglycerin.

The manuscripts may be submitted in German or English language. The papers are not allowed already to be published or only during 2002 and 2003, nor to have already won a prize. Since it is usual to include the prize-winning study in the symposium book, the authors by submitting their work they agree to its publication in full or in part (abstract).

An independent board of three well-known leading scientists will decide on behalf of the donor Pohl-Boskamp on the award of the Nitrolingual Prize. The price consists of an endowed amount of DM 10,000 and a medal.

The Nitrolingual Prize will be awarded on the 10th Hamburg Nitroglycerin Symposium 2003. Studies should be sent by registered mail to the address of the donor: G. Pohl-Boskamp GmbH & Co., Kieler Str. 11, P.O. Box 80, D-25551 Hohenlockstedt.

Closing date is 1st February 2003.

Bei Fragen zur Produktsicherheit wenden Sie sich bitte an:
If you have any questions regarding product safety,
please contact:

Walter de Gruyter GmbH
Genthiner Straße 13
10785 Berlin
productsafety@degruyterbrill.com